# Disaster Response for Beef Cattle Operations

*Editors*

CHRISTINE B. NAVARRE
DANIEL U. THOMSON

## VETERINARY CLINICS OF NORTH AMERICA: FOOD ANIMAL PRACTICE

www.vetfood.theclinics.com

*Consulting Editor*
ROBERT A. SMITH

July 2018 • Volume 34 • Number 2

**ELSEVIER**

1600 John F. Kennedy Boulevard ● Suite 1800 ● Philadelphia, Pennsylvania, 19103-2899

http://www.vetfood.theclinics.com

**VETERINARY CLINICS OF NORTH AMERICA: FOOD ANIMAL PRACTICE Volume 34, Number 2**
**July 2018 ISSN 0749-0720, ISBN-13: 978-0-323-61299-9**

Editor: Colleen Dietzler
Developmental Editor: Meredith Madeira

*Veterinary Clinics of North America: Food Animal Practice* (ISSN 0749-0720) is published in March, July, and November by Elsevier Inc., 360 Park Avenue South, New York, NY 10010-1710. Subscription prices are $250.00 per year (domestic individuals), $413.00 per year (domestic institutions), $100.00 per year (domestic students/residents), $276.00 per year (Canadian individuals), $545.00 per year (Canadian institutions), $335.00 per year (international individuals), $545.00 per year (international institutions), and $165.00 per year (international and Canadian students/residents). To receive student/resident rate, orders must be accompanied by name of affiliated institution, date of term, and the signature of program/residency coordinator on institution letterhead. *Clinics* subscription prices. All prices are subject to change without notice. **POSTMASTER:** Send address changes to *Veterinary Clinics of North America: Food Animal Practice*, Elsevier Health Sciences Division, Subscription Customer Service, 3251 Riverport Lane, Maryland Heights, MO 63043. Customer Service (orders, claims, online, change of address): Elsevier Health Sciences Division, Subscription **Customer Service, 3251 Riverport Lane, Maryland Heights, MO 63043. Tel: 1-800-654-2452 (U.S. and Canada); 314-447-8871 (ouside U.S. and Canada). Fax: 314-447-8029. E-mail: journalscustomerservice-usa@elsevier.com (for print support); journalsonlinesupport-usa@elsevier.com (for online support).**

*Reprints.* For copies of 100 or more, of articles in this publication, please contact the Commercial Reprints Department, Elsevier Inc., 360 Park Avenue South, New York, NY 10010-1710. Tel.: 212-633-3874; Fax: 212-633-3820; E-mail: reprints@elsevier.com.

*Veterinary Clinics of North America: Food Animal Practice* is covered in *Current Contents/Agriculture, Biology and Environmental Sciences, MEDLINE/PubMed (Index Medicus),* and *Excerpta Medica.*

# Contributors

## CONSULTING EDITOR

**ROBERT A. SMITH, DVM, MS**
Diplomate, American Board of Veterinary Practitioners; Veterinary Research and
Consulting Services, LLC, Greeley, Colorado, USA

## EDITORS

**CHRISTINE B. NAVARRE, DVM, MS**
Diplomate, American College of Veterinary Internal Medicine; Extension Veterinarian,
LSU AgCenter, Professor, School of Animal Sciences, Louisiana State University,
Baton Rouge, Louisiana, USA

**DANIEL U. THOMSON, PhD, DVM**
Jones Professor of Production Medicine, Kansas State University, College of Veterinary
Medicine, Manhattan, Kansas, USA

## AUTHORS

**DANELLE A. BICKETT-WEDDLE, DVM, MPH, PhD**
Diplomate, American College of Veterinary Preventive Medicine; Associate Director,
Center for Food Security and Public Health, Iowa State University, Ames, Iowa, USA

**WESLEY BISSETT Jr, DVM, PhD**
Associate Professor and Director, Texas A&M Veterinary Emergency Team, Large Animal
Clinical Sciences, Texas A&M University Veterinary Medicine & Biomedical Sciences,
College Station, Texas, USA

**SAMANTHA L. BOYAJIAN, BS**
College of Veterinary Medicine, Kansas State University, Manhattan, Kansas, USA

**SCOTT E. COTTON, MS, CPRM**
Area Educator, University of Wyoming Extension, Casper, Wyoming, USA

**RUSS DALY, DVM, MS**
Diplomate, American College of Veterinary Preventive Medicine; Extension Veterinarian/
Professor, State Public Health Veterinarian, Department of Veterinary and Biomedical
Science, South Dakota State University, Brookings, South Dakota, USA

**JOANNA DAVIS, DVM**
Emergency Coordinator for Georgia Florida, USDA APHIS Veterinary Services,
Surveillance, Preparedness, and Response Services (SPRS), Conyers, Georgia, USA

**RENÉE DAWN DEWELL, DVM, MS**
Veterinary Specialist, Department of Veterinary Microbiology and Preventive Medicine,
Center for Food Security and Public Health, Iowa State University, Ames, Iowa, USA

**DEE ELLIS, DVM, MPA**
Veterinarian, Institute for Infectious Animal Diseases (IIAD), Texas A&M University System, College Station, Texas, USA

**CYNTHIA MARSHALL FAUX, DVM, PhD**
Diplomate, American College of Veterinary Internal Medicine - Large Animal; Clinical Assistant Professor, Department of Integrated Physiology and Neurosciences, Washington State University College of Veterinary Medicine, Washington State University, Pullman, Washington, USA

**DAVID P. GNAD, DVM, MS**
Nebraska Veterinary Services, West Point, Nebraska, USA

**DEE GRIFFIN, DVM, MS**
Director, Texas A&M Veterinary Medical Center, West Texas A&M University, Canyon, Texas, USA

**CARLA HUSTON, DVM, PhD**
Associate Professor, Department of Pathobiology and Population Medicine, Mississippi State University College of Veterinary Medicine, Mississippi State, Mississippi, USA

**ARTHUR LEE JONES, DVM, MS**
Associate Professor, Department of Population Health, UGA College of Veterinary Medicine, Tifton, Georgia, USA

**JOHN L. KELLENBERGER, DVM**
Ashland Veterinary Center, Ashland, Kansas, USA

**NELS N. LINDBERG, DVM**
Production Animal Consultation, Great Bend, Kansas, USA

**TERRY L. MADER, MS, PhD**
Professor Emeritus, University of Nebraska, Mader Consulting LLC, Gretna, Nebraska, USA

**REBECCA McCONNICO, DVM, PhD**
Professor and Veterinarian, School of Agricultural Sciences and Forestry, College of Applied and Natural Sciences, Louisiana Tech University, Ruston, Louisiana, USA

**CHRISTINE B. NAVARRE, DVM, MS**
Diplomate, American College of Veterinary Internal Medicine; Extension Veterinarian, LSU AgCenter, Professor, School of Animal Sciences, Louisiana State University, Baton Rouge, Louisiana, USA

**K.C. OLSON, MS, PhD**
Professor, Department of Animal Sciences and Industry, Kansas State University, Manhattan, Kansas, USA

**ELIZABETH J. PARKER, DVM**
International and Strategic Partnerships Specialist, AgriLife Research, Texas A&M University, College Station, Texas, USA

**LISA PEDERSON, M.Agr**
Extension Beef Quality Specialist, North Dakota State University Extension Service, Dickinson Research Extension Center, Bismarck, North Dakota, USA

**DAVID N. RETHORST, DVM**
Beef Health Solutions, Wamego, Kansas, USA

**MICHAEL W. SANDERSON, DVM, MS**
Diplomate, American College of Veterinary Preventive Medicine (Epidemiology Specialty); Professor, Epidemiology and Beef Production, Center for Outcomes Research and Epidemiology, Kansas State University, Manhattan, Kansas, USA

**JAN K. SHEARER, DVM, MS**
Professor and Extension Veterinarian, Department of Veterinary Diagnostic and Production Animal Medicine, College of Veterinary Medicine, Iowa State University, Ames, Iowa, USA

**DAVID B. SJEKLOCHA, DVM**
Operations Manager, Animal Health and Welfare, Cattle Empire LLC, Satanta, Kansas, USA

**RANDALL K. SPARE, DVM**
Ashland Veterinary Center, Ashland, Kansas, USA

**KEVIN F. SULLIVAN, BVSc**
Principle Veterinarian, Bell Veterinary Services, Queensland, Australia

**JIMMY TICKEL, DVM**
Northeastern Region EP Veterinarian, North Carolina Department of Agriculture and Consumer Services, Raleigh, North Carolina, USA

**JUSTIN W. WAGGONER, MS, PhD**
Associate Professor, Southwest Research and Extension Center, Kansas State University, Garden City, Kansas, USA

**ERIN WASSON, BSW, MSW, RSW**
Clinical Associate Social Work, Veterinary Social Work Program, Western College of Veterinary Medicine, University of Saskatchewan, Saskatchewan, Canada

**AUDRY WIEMAN, DVM**
Ridgeline Vet Services, LLC, Lynch, Nebraska, USA

**JERRY YATES, BS**
Farm Manager, Reymann Memorial Farms, Beef Quality Assurance Collaborator, West Virginia University Davis College of Agriculture, Wardensville, West Virginia, USA

# Contents

**Preface: Responding to Natural Disasters and Emergencies in Beef Production**     xiii

Christine B. Navarre and Daniel U. Thomson

**Communication and Working with Authorities During Natural Disasters**     223

Dee Ellis, Rebecca McConnico, and Jimmy Tickel

Keeping people and animals out of harm's way, preventing property loss, and working together in the community with other animal stakeholders and officials are important in building community resilience during disasters. Developing plans for neighbors helping each other evacuate animals is important. Producer helping producer, veterinarian helping veterinarian, and community helping community build resilience by preventing loss, responding to needs, and recovering and restoring livelihoods.

**Cattle Assessment On-Site During Emergencies**     233

Arthur Lee Jones, Renée Dawn Dewell, and Joanna Davis

Veterinary assessment of the condition and needs of livestock and their owners in an emergency is an essential element of the disaster response. The emergency response for livestock has 4 critical components: assessing the need for and attending to the immediate medical needs of injured or affected livestock; determining the resources available to meet the needs, including feed and facilities; identifying any ongoing threats or potential hazards to livestock health and welfare; and appropriate documentation of damages and actions by responders. Information gathered from cattle assessments by veterinarians is used to prioritize resources and plan for anticipated needs.

**Feeding and Watering Beef Cattle During Disasters**     249

Justin W. Waggoner and K.C. Olson

Animal care, feeding, and nutrition in the wake of a natural disaster or emergency situation are difficult and require resourcefulness. Immediately following the event, the most basic needs essential for survival of cattle (ie, water, feed, rest, and recovery) should be addressed. Once these basic needs have been addressed, the primary objective then becomes to maintain the present condition of the animals to reduce the potential for negative production outcomes. This article provides a general overview of feeding and managing cattle immediately following a natural disaster or emergency situation.

**Tornado Preparation and Response in Feedlot Cattle**     259

Samantha L. Boyajian, Nels N. Lindberg, and David P. Gnad

Encouraging operations to develop emergency protocols is one of the best steps one can take as a veterinarian who may be called upon to help once disaster strikes. Poor plans yield slow progress, and in times of tornado damage, efficiency in recovery is critical for an operation. A veterinarian is a key player in animal stewardship as well as human health and safety during natural disasters.

**Blizzards and Range Cattle: Management Before, During, and After the Storm**     265

Russ Daly and Cynthia Marshall Faux

Numerous factors contribute to the outcome and recovery for range cattle affected by blizzard. Consequences and impact on the producer depend on the timing of the storm relative to the herd's production cycle, access to shelter, duration and intensity of the storm, and poststorm emergency management. Critical planning efforts by the producer include clear animal identification methods, identification of sheltering options, and consideration of animal indemnity and insurance requirements. Including range animals in local and state disaster planning efforts facilitates response and recovery efforts. Response efforts must include understanding of postincident animal behavior concerns and producer and responder mental health.

**Management of Confined Cattle in Blizzard Conditions**     277

David B. Sjeklocha

Preparation and prioritization are essential to managing confined cattle through a severe winter storm. Water, feed, and cattle comfort are the top priorities for cattle after a blizzard, and making sure employees understand those priorities and how to address them will help to minimize cattle stress and losses.

**Wildfire Response in Range Cattle**     281

David N. Rethorst, Randall K. Spare, and John L. Kellenberger

The manner in which the producers and communities affected by the Starbuck fire dealt with the aftermath and recovery is the focus of this article. Ranchers, as stewards of the cattle, had to assess and attend to the welfare of survivors, euthanize the severally damaged, dispose of the dead, and deal with inadequate federal assistance and insurance claims. Veterinarians acted as coordinators of the community relief effort and supported the ranchers. The practical and psychological effects, and more humane possible future scenarios, are described.

**Preparation and Response to Truck Accidents on Highways Involving Cattle**     289

Lisa Pederson, Jerry Yates, and Audry Wieman

Annually, in the United States, more than 50 million head of cattle are transported. Most are transported via semitrailer. As the number of livestock transported via motor vehicles has increased, so has the number of accidents involving livestock transport. Most livestock transport accidents in the United States involved semitrailers carrying cattle. Before the Bovine Emergency Response Program, no standard operating procedures existed for accidents involving livestock transport in the United States. The Bovine Emergency Response Plan provides a framework for veterinarians, emergency responders, and law enforcement to better address accidents involving cattle transport.

**Preparation and Response for Flooding Events in Beef Cattle**    309

Wesley Bissett Jr, Carla Huston, and Christine B. Navarre

Flooding seems to be occurring at an increased frequency and severity, resulting in significant losses to the beef cattle industry. Responding to the needs of beef cattle is a resource-intense occurrence and beyond that provided by most local jurisdictions. It is incumbent on livestock producers to develop continuity of operations or emergency plans designed to limit the financial losses and compromised animal welfare that occur when livestock are exposed to flood conditions. Livestock producers and the veterinary medical profession should also encourage and participate in the development of public emergency plans focused on limiting losses in this critical industry.

**Managing Heat Stress Episodes in Confined Cattle**    325

Kevin F. Sullivan and Terry L. Mader

Feedlot cattle consuming large amounts of feed and gaining weight rapidly generate significant amounts of metabolic heat. In summer, failure to dissipate this heat leads to heat accumulation and heat stress. Respiratory rates, panting scores, and behavioral changes are useful indicators of heat stress in cattle. Ceasing cattle movement, providing supplementary water tanks in the pens, cooling the pen surface, and manipulation of nutrition and feeding management should be considered to mitigate the risk and manage a heat stress crisis. Removing manure from the pens and provisions of shade have been found to be beneficial for cattle exposed to hot climates.

**Foreign Animal Disease Outbreaks**    341

Danelle A. Bickett-Weddle, Michael W. Sanderson, and Elizabeth J. Parker

A foreign animal disease (FAD) infecting beef cattle can have a negative impact on producers and the veterinarians who serve them. A veterinarian's ability to recognize FADs is a significant responsibility, as is aiding clients and local community in preparing for and responding to an outbreak. Knowledge of local livestock operations, markets, and resources provides valuable insight to managing officials and speeds response. Business continuity for clients and veterinarians will be affected by movement controls. Successful control and eradication of an FAD requires a concerted effort by producers, veterinarians, emergency responders, and state and federal officials.

**Humane Euthanasia and Carcass Disposal**    355

Jan K. Shearer, Dee Griffin, and Scott E. Cotton

Euthanasia is ending life in a way that minimizes or eliminates pain and distress. It requires techniques that induce loss of consciousness followed by cardiac and respiratory arrest and loss of brain function. Although euthanasia is the objective for uncontrollable animal suffering, it is not always possible. Euthanasia of animals using barbiturates or barbituric acid derivatives is impractical for situations that require mass euthanasia of multiple animals. Selection of the most appropriate disposal method depends on number of carcasses, potential environmental impact, climatic conditions, and other factors. Preplanning and training are requirements for proper application of euthanasia procedures and disposal of carcasses.

**Mental Health During Environmental Crisis and Mass Incident Disasters** 375

Erin Wasson and Audry Wieman

Veterinarians responding to animal health-related incidents are in the same class as first responders and should be aware of similar mental health concerns. Cultivating resiliency, identifying symptoms, and linking individuals to support systems are practical strategies to provide positive outcomes for veterinarians facing difficult experiences. This article explores veterinarians as first responders and farm stress and provides an overview of mental health responses to trauma; strategies and interventions for individuals, families, communities, and veterinarians; a discussion of boundaries and threshold for managing crisis; barriers and considerations for service provision; and a summary and discussion of future research and curriculum opportunities.

# VETERINARY CLINICS OF NORTH AMERICA: FOOD ANIMAL PRACTICE

**FORTHCOMING ISSUES**

*November 2018*
**Mastitis**
Pamela L. Ruegg and
Christina Petersson-Wolfe, *Editors*

*March 2019*
**Housing and Environment Issues of Dairy Cattle**
Nigel Cook, *Editor*

*July 2019*
**Fetal Programming and Epigenetics**
Rick Funston, *Editor*

**RECENT ISSUES**

*March 2018*
**Digestive Disorders of the Abomasum and Intestines**
Robert J. Callan and Meredyth L. Jones, *Editors*

*November 2017*
**Digestive Disorders of the Forestomach**
Robert J. Callan and Meredyth Jones, *Editors*

*July 2017*
**Lameness in Cattle**
J.K. Shearer, *Editor*

**RELATED INTEREST**

Feedlot Processing and Arrival Cattle Management, July 2015
Brad J. White, Daniel U. Thomson, *Editors*

**THE CLINICS ARE NOW AVAILABLE ONLINE!**
Access your subscription at:
www.theclinics.com

# Preface

# Responding to Natural Disasters and Emergencies in Beef Production

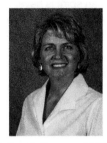 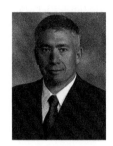

Christine B. Navarre, DVM, MS     Daniel U. Thomson, PhD, DVM
*Editors*

On March 7, 2017, the Starbuck Wildfire occurred on the Kansas and Oklahoma border. The city of Ashland, Kansas had to be evacuated, and a total of 833,966 acres were lost to the fire. People lost their lives, lost their homes, and lost their livestock, horses, and companion animals in the fire. The Ashland Veterinary Clinic served as the command center for farmers, ranchers, and community members. Thousands of firefighters, medical first responders, police, highway patrol, the Army National Guard, and many other volunteers came to this area to serve those in need. After Dr Thomson watched the volunteer veterinarians in the area of the Starbuck Wildfire deal with that disaster, it was clear that something was needed to help prepare and respond to the next natural disaster.

There is quite a bit of information available on responding to natural disasters. However, to our knowledge, no one has ever put together a series of veterinary articles written by people that have firsthand experience and emergency response training specifically for beef cattle veterinarians. Dr Thomson solicited the help of Dr Christine Navarre and Dr Bob Smith, and this issue was born.

As we made our list of topics, we thought about our colleagues, friends, producers, and people who had expertise in these areas from firsthand experience to extensive training in food animal rescue and medicine. Each article partners veterinarians from private practice, academia, and government organizations to bring practical, straightforward guidance on natural disasters. We are thankful for the great response and expertise that volunteered to complete this issue of *Veterinary Clinics of North America: Food Animal Practice*.

The American Veterinary Medical Association states on their Web site, "The AVMA encourages veterinary professionals in all facets of public, private, and government

Vet Clin Food Anim 34 (2018) xiii–xiv
https://doi.org/10.1016/j.cvfa.2018.04.001
0749-0720/18/© 2018 Published by Elsevier Inc.

**vetfood.theclinics.com**

sectors to communicate and participate with their local and state emergency management organizations to ensure that veterinary medical resources are integrated in emergency management plans. Disaster planning should encompass the "all animals–all hazards" philosophy and include mitigation, preparedness, response, and recovery."

Preparedness works. We encourage veterinarians to work with their community, state, and national leaders to prepare and train for these emergencies. Veterinarians should prepare their families and their practices and help their clients prepare. We hope that this issue offers some practical advice on preparedness, and when that fails, better tools to respond.

Unfortunately, natural disasters happen. However, the American spirit is never seen so beautifully than in a time of need. Veterinarians are a pillar of unsung heroes in our communities. Our animals and food supply depend on these unsung heroes in times of need like those discussed in this issue.

Christine B. Navarre, DVM, MS
LSU AgCenter
School of Animal Sciences
Louisiana State University
111 Dalrymple Building
110 LSU Union Square
Baton Rouge, LA 70803-0106, USA

Daniel U. Thomson, PhD, DVM
Kansas State University
College of Veterinary Medicine
1800 Denison Avenue
Manhattan, KS 66506, USA

*E-mail addresses:*
CNavarre@agcenter.lsu.edu (C.B. Navarre)
dthomson@vet.k-state.edu (D.U. Thomson)

# Communication and Working with Authorities During Natural Disasters

Dee Ellis, DVM, MPA[a],*, Rebecca McConnico, DVM, PhD[b,c], Jimmy Tickel, DVM[d]

## KEYWORDS

- Communication • Natural disasters • Working with authorities

## KEY POINTS

- Keeping people and animals out of harm's way, preventing property loss, and working together in the community with animal health officials, other animal agriculture stakeholders and officials are important in building community resilience during disasters.
- Developing plans for neighbors helping each other evacuate animals is important.
- Producer helping producer, veterinarian helping veterinarian, and community helping community build resilience by preventing loss, responding to needs, and recovering and restoring livelihoods.

## INTRODUCTION

During natural disasters, veterinarians may be simultaneously a victim, a veterinarian for their own clients' animals, and a first responder dealing with other animal issues. This complex mix of obligations and risks makes it critical that veterinarians not only have a plan for disasters but also understand who their plans will interdict. That forward-facing duty as a veterinary practitioner is the focus of this article, which explores the plans and links with infrastructure that veterinarians can put in place to help mitigate disasters involving beef cattle.

## WHO IS IN CHARGE?

In preparing for this article, numerous first-responder veterinary officials were queried (Jeff Turner, Texas Animal Health Commission, Emergency Management Coordinator,

The authors have nothing to disclose.
[a] Institute for Infectious Animal Diseases (IIAD), Texas A&M University System, 1500 Research Parkway, Suite B270, College Station, TX 77845, USA; [b] School of Agricultural Sciences, College of Applied and Natural Sciences, Louisiana Tech University, 1501 Reese Drive, Ruston, LA 71270, USA; [c] Forestry, College of Applied and Natural Sciences, Louisiana Tech University, 1501 Reese Drive, Ruston, LA 71270, USA; [d] North Carolina Department of Agriculture and Consumer Services, 2 W Edenton Street, Raleigh, NC 27601, USA
* Corresponding author.
E-mail address: Dee.Ellis@ag.tamu.edu

Vet Clin Food Anim 34 (2018) 223–232
https://doi.org/10.1016/j.cvfa.2018.03.003
0749-0720/18/© 2018 Elsevier Inc. All rights reserved.

vetfood.theclinics.com

personal communication, January 5, 2018; Greg Christy, DVM, Emergency Programs Veterinarian Manager, Division of Animal Industry, Florida Department of Agriculture and Consumer Services, personal communication, January 4, 2018; Nick Striegel, DVM, MPH, Colorado Assistant State Veterinarian, Colorado Department of Agriculture, Animal Health Division, personal communication, January 5, 2018; Kent Fowler, DVM, Animal Health Branch Chief, California Department of Food and Agriculture, personal communication, January 3, 2018; Grant Miller, DVM, Director of Regulatory Affairs, California Veterinary Medical Association, personal communication, January 5, 2018)[1] about what the message should be for practicing veterinarians whose clinic or clients are involved in a disaster occurrence. The resounding answer was for veterinarians to "engage" before an event with all the authorities and resources they may encounter or need during a disaster. Although volunteers are always needed during a situation, being engaged and prepared before simply spontaneously volunteering when an incident unfolds has obvious advantages that will be clearly delineated in the following pages.

The most effective responses on behalf of livestock in disasters occur in states and counties/parishes where industry and government have formed a relationship before the event. Veterinarians are an integral part of these relationships and can get involved at many levels. They should be familiar with the myriad of people, organizations, and government entities that they may encounter during a disaster event.

### Local Responders

Livestock response plans vary from location to location, so understanding who oversees livestock issues during nondisaster days as well as during disasters is important to help producers and veterinarians know who would be most helpful during an emergency. At the county or parish level, first responders routinely involved in an animal response include the county emergency management staff, county extension personnel, sheriff's department, animal control officials, agriculture teachers, and local volunteer organizations. These people would attend planning meetings and assist in the role of animal first responders. In many states, these county level response personnel are organized into a group and titled the County Animal Response Team (CART). Veterinarians in the county are valuable members of a county CART.

### Emergency managers

Emergency manager (EM) officials are the gatekeepers to all official emergency response in the county or parish. They coordinate the first responder community actions and are the number one source of information before and during disaster situations. They are often overwhelmed with human issues and welcome support from other stakeholders on animal issues. If a veterinarian does not know where to start in learning more about the local disaster response plans for animals, any county official can point them in the right direction.

### Cooperative extension

Extension service personnel involvement and resources vary across states. They are great resources to those areas that have them. County extension officials often play a lead role in managing any local animal response plans, whether it involves leadership in a CART, or shelter, or supply point that is receiving donated feed/hay. Veterinarians interested in local disaster response should get acquainted with their county extension officials.

### Animal control officials

Animal control agencies are the officials responsible for animals in local communities. Although they may not be working directly with livestock during disasters, animal control officials may have information about stray or injured livestock and can facilitate needs for gathering, rescuing, sheltering, or feeding in place.

### Cattle industry stakeholders
Many disaster experiences have proven that by far the best resource a cattle owner has in an emergency is another cattle owner! No one has more local knowledge than a rancher when there are decisions to be made about accessing stranded cattle, or the best way to distribute hay and feed to those in need. Cattle growers, cattle associations, and cattle industry support personnel own and operate most resources and expertise needed to respond to on behalf of impacted cattle owners. In some states, local ranchers will be imbedded formally in local response efforts as "liaisons" for emergency responders assigned to an incident.

### Command post
Representatives of state cattlemen associations may do the same at agriculture (multi-agency coordinating centers [MACC] or state Emergency Operations Center [EOC]) locations in many states.

### State Veterinarian and Commissioner/Secretary of Agriculture or Animal Health Commissioner
State officials are often the strongest advocates for cattle growers regarding disaster response and recovery because they are also tasked with preparing for disease issues that require substantial amounts of response planning. State level officials speak for the industry regarding assistance programs on both the state and the federal level and can seek declarations that will benefit producers in large disaster events. Most often, assistance for lost animals, repairs to farm property, and mortality management are coordinated by state officials with funding from United States Department of Agriculture (USDA), often as part of an MACC. Assistance from well-known sources such as Federal Emergency Management System (FEMA) are usually reserved for response to those impacts affecting humans, but there are times that FEMA funds may be used for animal issues that impact human health or safety.

### Other law enforcement agencies
State agency rangers and fire brand inspectors are part of natural disaster response plans in many states. They can support supply point and feed/hay distribution and security if needed, but also play a pivotal role in ensuring stray cattle are identified and returned to the owner. Just like in their "normal job," they also ensure cattle are not stolen during disaster events. These officials are often certified peace officers and are also critical to maintaining public safety and protecting public property (including cattle) in disasters.

### State emergency management agencies
All states have emergency management agencies that are structured to complement the federal response structure. There may be many different agencies or authorities involved in the various animal response activities within an overall response depending on the state.

### State animal response teams
**State Farm Bureau** Farm Bureau livestock committees may assist in disaster response. For example, in Louisiana, Farm Bureau members are involved in matching up hay donations with requests for hay for livestock.

**Nongovernment volunteer response groups** Volunteer response organizations may be brought into disaster situations to assist the official response efforts or may appear on scene without being invited. Groups that have an MOU/MOA (Memorandum of Understanding/Memorandum of Agreement) or contract and that have been invited and specifically tasked are most desired because they will not only be part of an organized plan and effort but also will be supported by the response. As an example, a properly activated livestock rescue group will know where to conduct rescue operations as well as where to transport animals for shelter or where to seek veterinary care if needed. In some larger cities and towns, it is becoming more common for some agreements/contracts to be setup between civil jurisdiction and volunteer nongovernmental organizations (NGOs) because it can be more efficient to address urgent issues without having to go through the state level administration.

### Veterinary response teams

Many veterinary schools and NGOs also have volunteer veterinary units. These units may be very well organized and staffed with veterinarians, technicians, and triage equipment. They will routinely be working under the umbrella of the state entity in charge of animal response. Working with the state authorities will ensure they are licensed, trained, vetted, credentialed, and aware of all state and local obligations expected by the appropriate state response agency.

**State Veterinary Medical Associations** Veterinary Medical Associations have become more and more involved in animal disaster response and planning, and many have emergency response committees. They assist in state policy decisions for veterinary volunteers related to licensure reciprocity with the appropriate state licensing boards and can assist in coordinating veterinary response. California, for example, has the largest volunteer veterinary response capability in the United States, with more than 1500 veterinary volunteers enrolled in the California Veterinary Medical Reserve Core. This entity is under the auspices of the California Veterinary Medical Association and assists veterinarians with both training and credentialing opportunities related to animal health and public health.[2]

### Federal Responders

If a disaster declaration has worked its way up the ladder of scope from county judge/manager to the Governor to the Presidential level, veterinarians may work with federal agency personnel. At the community level, they are often fewer than similar state personnel and often have very specific functions.

### United States Department of Agriculture

USDA under its Emergency Support Function (ESF 11) responsibility will have the most field personnel deployed in major animal disasters situations.[3] USDA agencies that may routinely respond include the following:

1. Veterinary services: often assist state animal health officials with a variety of issues
2. Animal care: evaluates facilities with captive animals such as zoos that may be affected
3. Wildlife services: may assist with either wildlife issues or in evaluating locations of stranded livestock by helicopter and even delivering feed by helicopter in some states
4. National Resources Conservation Service: may assist with debris management, including carcass disposal

### Department of the Interior, Bureau of Land Management

Many western states have cattle grazing on "public" land. The Department of the Interior, Bureau of Land Management is instrumental in response efforts if a wildfire impacted cattle grazing on federal public lands.

### American Veterinary Medical Association

The American Veterinary Medical Association (AVMA) has been a leader in veterinary emergency response planning and response over the years. A myriad of valuable resources for veterinary planning and response can be found on the AVMA Disaster Preparedness for Veterinarians Web page.[4]

## PLANNING

Veterinarians are inherently one of the occupations with the highest levels of trust by the community. Strengthening the trust between first responders and cattlemen who may be reluctant or too proud to accept help is beneficial for public safety and animal well-being during a disaster. Bovine practitioners can provide leadership for community planning by hosting a meeting where rancher clients can become acquainted with local officials and engage together in planning discussions. Such meetings could provide a real boost to local planning and readiness, while strengthening client bases and clinic loyalty.

Being engaged in planning efforts has other important benefits. It may increase the likelihood of a veterinarian being reimbursed for any services offered during a disaster. Preexisting contracts (or agreements) can in certain situations be signed between county officials and potential responders, including veterinarians. Although there are less federal/state/county funding reimbursements available for cattle situations than horses or pet animal response activities, there are still opportunities. Whether the expense is shelter/boarding, feeding, veterinary care, or veterinary consulting, the first step in exploring the possibilities for reimbursement should be with the county emergency management coordinator. If displaced cattle are "dropped off" by well-meaning citizens at a veterinary clinic pen, another possibility for reimbursement for feed and housing costs of those animals may be through the state "estray" laws. Veterinarians should discuss pre-contracts for response support and housing strays with county officials.

Veterinarians/clinics that have preexisting contracts and credentialing and are part of the county response plan-in-advance allow a clinic potential access to resources that may otherwise be unavailable if requested on the spur of the moment during an event. These resources may help a clinic reopen quicker, which saves response resources and brings normality back to a community.

### Personal/Farm/Ranch/Veterinary Clinic Readiness

One of the most common observations that practitioners report after a natural disaster has occurred is personal family suffering because they could not close their clinic because client animals were still there and needed care. Family planning should come first, meaning a clinic plan must be in place allowing for closing when appropriate. Once a veterinarian has personal and clinic emergency plans, they can become involved in operations working with first responders, general public, and clients during a disaster situation.

Veterinarians can play a key role in helping their clients prepare a farm/ranch readiness plan. For more information on planning at the farm/ranch level, please see Wesley Bissett and colleagues' article, "Flooding," in this issue.

Personal ranch/farm/clinic readiness includes communicating to local officials (first responder groups, EMs, county/parish extension, and animal control) direct knowledge of individual farm/ranch/clinic situations and emergency plans (number/ type of animals, animal identification, resources for moving animals, and so forth). Personal communication between local veterinarians and first responders will optimize the chances that farm/ranch/clinic is in a position to receive assistance.

Included in an effective farm/ranch/clinic readiness plan is a detailed map that illustrates the location of cattle (and other animals), a few pictures of cattle/animal type, as well as pictures of brands or tags used. Providing detailed information will facilitate more effective interactions with community disaster assistance operations.

### Training

Responders in the United States follow the Incident Command System (ICS) structure for organized response. A veterinarian would be well served to learn the basics of this system. There are online courses offered by FEMA for ICS 100 and the National Incident Management System 700 course. In just 2 hours, a veterinarian can learn the basics of how any emergency response is organized at the local or higher levels. There are similar courses often offered in person for county level or volunteer organization personnel, or through veterinary associations. Some of the courses may qualify for continuing education credits.

### Credentialing

Besides the advantages of potential reimbursement contracts put in place before an event, and training aspects that could include continuing education opportunities, there may be credentialing available to responding veterinarians preengaged in the planning process. "Credentialed responders" performing an approved task may be able to access gasoline at government supply points not available to the public, and entrance to areas otherwise secure from the public to treat or evaluate.

### Communication

Staying in touch during a disaster is critical, and a communications plan is essential. Disasters vary in how they affect the ability to communicate, especially for ranchers/ producers. In many areas impacted by large events such as hurricanes, modern methods of communication may remain intact and help can be a cell phone call or e-mail away. In other situations, as demonstrated in Hurricanes Katrina, Rita, Irma, and Maria, communication can be severely impacted. Thus, consideration for redundancy of communication methods when developing response plans, including telephone, e-mail, text messaging, social media, or standard media, is essential. Family members, ranch/farm personnel, and veterinary clinic staff should have access to different brands and types of devices (telephones/laptops) and reliable cellular service carriers. Experience has shown that some will work better than others in disasters.

Overall, response officials on both state and county/parish levels will attempt to coordinate information that would go to producers and make this information available by all the above-mentioned methods. Even so, there may be times just after disasters that all communication fails and so planning needs to account for actions that would be taken in the event communication fails. These preplanned actions would include activities such as preplanned opening of designated resource staging sites where producers would know that even without communications, they could not only receive needed items such as feed but also provide and receive information and guidance as to what needs to be done and what currently is being done on behalf of livestock and their owners.

Up-to-date contact lists on devices are critical. Having extended family or friends listed as an emergency contact in farm or veterinary clinic plans and elsewhere is advised. Designation of someone outside the affected area who can fill in as a proxy secretary for a producer or veterinary clinic until service is reestablished in the area will allow problem solving and continuity of operations to be more efficient. This option is critical in situations where the ranch owners' telephone resources have become damaged (eg, water damage, loss) because replacement telephones may not readily available. A communications proxy needs to have knowledge and details of this responsibility, which may be over an extended period of time. Identifying representatives (including government officials and industry representatives) who can provide a voice on behalf of the cattle industry is also important.

### Satellite phones
Although expensive, satellite phones can be quite useful in disasters, and so, an association or producer group might consider the need to purchase such a device. (It is recommended to consult your local EM before investing in such technology.)

### Ham radio
Ham radio operators have proven useful in many disasters and can be helpful to cattlemen if they are known. Contacting and coordination with local emergency coordinators are critical because this communication option is often already included as a local resource. Ham operator communications were used extensively in the 2017 hurricanes.

### Landline telephone
Landline telephones are reliable when local telephone lines are uninterrupted. They are "constant" connections because power outages will not affect landline telephone service. There is added safety because 911 operators can determine exact locations automatically from a landline. Landlines rarely "drop" a telephone call, and most are included in the local telephone book, and other hard copy or Internet directories.

### Cell phone
Mobile phones are a must for everyone now. An opportunity to stay in touch with friends and family members during disaster situations (small or large scale) is important and allows access to e-mail, business associates, and emergency responders. In addition, smart phone technologies, including picture capabilities, allow for quicker field assessments to be made. Telephones with push-to-talk features worked very well during Hurricanes Katrina and Rita when most cell phone towers were damaged. Text messaging has proven to be the most reliable form of electronic communication in many disasters.

### Two-way radios
Two-way radios do not rely on telephone lines, electricity (except to charge the batteries), or towers. They transmit messages as far as 12 miles in optimal conditions. They allow for regular voice communication and require no special training or expensive equipment. A set of 2-way radios is a critical component of a home or business disaster kit.

### Social media networking tools
Tools such as Twitter and Facebook can be used in a variety of ways to support emergency management and public health and safety. Despite there being some concerns about lack of expression of relevant information and questionable data quality, there is no doubt that the information landscape is changing. Millennials are embracing social media like no generation before, and older generations also realize the importance of being connected using these communication tools. Engagement between the private and government sectors on how social media tools might serve as a conduit for 2-way

communication locally with EMs and law enforcement officials to improve local and regional recovery decision making would be beneficial.

## E-mail

Home/farm and business communications through e-mail is one of the more important business applications. For many businesses, maintaining business continuity depends on e-mail continuity. A backup plan for loss of e-mail continuity is critical during disaster situations.

## Message boards

Electronic message boards are useful for communications and are a secondary means of trying to locate missing persons, animals, property, or as a means of obtaining additional information during disasters. In some cases, bulletin boards and simple posted messages may be the only means of communication. Both urban search and rescue and animal search and rescue teams use codes to indicate the results of a specific building or area search.

## On-Star alert system

On-Star alert system is a form of communication using more than just a 911-type call. Pushing the red button in a disaster or emergency situation will alert a trained advisor. These advisors have the capability of staying on the line until help arrives.

## RESPONSE
### Local

A disaster may or may not trigger an "emergency declaration." If it does, first the county EM declares an emergency. If the scope is affecting multiple counties, the Governor will declare a state emergency declaration followed by a federal declaration should the scope overwhelm state resources. The effect of these declarations is that they open avenues for outside personnel and funding to funnel into the community legally as well as allow waiver of normal rules and regulations that may deter timely response efforts.

Response components for large-scale disasters will include short- and long-term efforts and continuous communication support, such as the following:

1. Community assessment teams
2. Human and animal search and rescue: search-and-rescue and emergency medical responses often in environments wherein communication services are disrupted
3. Security and civil order: preserving civil order (eg, preventing looting) and ensuring public safety when everyday dispatch systems may be overloaded or inoperable; homes, businesses, and organizations should do their part on the local level to secure personal property, so community/civil law enforcement personnel are not overwhelmed.
4. Supply distribution: distributing food, water, and supplies for animals in addition to relief centers, coordinating and tracking inventory and shipments, and dispatching security for those centers
5. Relief coordination: coordinating the efforts of response (relief and rescue) workers and clean-up crews by communicating and tracking schedules and supply inventory.

It is important to understand that no matter how well prepared a local jurisdiction is for animal response, public safety and public health needs must come first. Animal disaster responders must be understanding in waiting for support, resources, or access to impacted areas. For example, if there are still search and rescue operations underway for people, animal response resources may be limited until that is over.

Animal control and extension are likely to be those called on to assist animals in emergencies, whereas law enforcement and emergency management will be the first to conduct assessments and surveys just after a disaster. Local jurisdictions will often have "shelters" established for displaced and evacuated animals. Displaced animals include captured strays loose on the roadways as well as animals evacuated to avoid harm. In both cases, a daily visit by a veterinary professional would be ideal to assist in evaluating the health and care of the animals housed. During the hurricanes of 2017 and those from the past, shelters had hundreds of dogs, horses, and other animals on the same premises (eg, cattle and small ruminants, poultry, exotics, reptiles, and companion animals).

Veterinarians and ranchers/owners must stay in tune with official weather reports, including the warnings and reports that would affect the timing of evacuation, sheltering, and other disaster-related operations. The National Oceanic Atmospheric Association Weather Radio All Hazards (NWR) is a nationwide network of radio stations broadcasting continuous weather information directly from the nearest National Weather Service office. NWR broadcasts official Weather Service warnings, watches, forecasts, and other hazard information 24 hours a day, 7 days a week (http://www.nws.noaa.gov/nwr/).

Feed and hay donations are one of the most difficult aspects of disaster response to manage. Requests for immediate needs often merge into a logistics nightmare. Social media can often prompt an overwhelming donation response. An official point of contact regarding donations should be designated ahead of time. A plan for donations management and supply delivery is critical, and in many states, donations are coordinated on the local level through emergency management using local resources such as cooperative extension and producer associations/groups (please see J.W. Waggoner and K.C. Olson's article, "Feeding and Watering Beef Cattle During Disasters," in this issue for more information on handling feed donations.)

## State

If county resources become overwhelmed, then state authorities will get involved. They may first be simply supporting the local resources in the early stages. Once multiple counties are involved, and/or a Governor's emergency declaration has been declared, there will start to be more state involvement and support to counties/parishes.

Most state level animal disaster issues are delegated from the state emergency management agency to a state agency with animal expertise. State agencies that are expected to manage animal disaster issues are often a state department of agriculture or the state animal health agency (if separate). Most but not all state veterinarian offices are housed within the state agriculture department. Bovine practitioners should familiarize themselves with the local representatives of their Department of Agriculture or State Veterinarian's office.

Besides supporting local responses, most state animal health officials will also be part of the overall state response for both *people* and *animals*. The Animal Health Agency for a state will almost always have a representative imbedded at the state Emergency Operation Center (EOC) with all other state agencies. Most of the activities at an EOC are people related, so the agriculture agency may also have their own standalone animal coordinating center. These centers are often called MACCs or agriculture EOCs. They could be as complex as actual facilities with representatives of all state agencies and stakeholders that deal with animals, or simply be a virtual setting that involves daily coordinating telephone calls. In almost every case, the agriculture MACC will include representatives of the Department of Agriculture, State

Veterinarian, State Extension, State Wildlife, veterinary response teams (if deployed), cattle/livestock associations, and veterinary medical associations. Animal responses are inherently multijurisdictional in nature. It is essential therefore that a veterinarian know as many know as many people involved in their respective local and state animal response activities as possible beforehand.

State authorities can assign volunteer resources and veterinary response teams to areas most in need of veterinary care and ensure that they get reimbursed for their services. State authorities can also ensure that volunteers do not accidentally or intentionally compete with local veterinary practitioners once they are open again. When the local veterinary infrastructure is open for business again, these resources can often be deployed elsewhere or demobilized.

Understanding the approach of official emergency management and Department of Agriculture/Health Commissions toward "at large livestock" provides owners/producers/practitioners a starting point for locating and identifying animals. Some states will market stray cattle, collecting information to provide sales proceeds to owners, whereas other states will attempt to shelter lost animals in locations designated in their county/parish or state response plans until claimed by owners. Information-sharing is critical for effective plans for animal identification and movement or livestock.

State veterinarians may need to seek permission from neighboring states for acceptance of displaced animals. In disasters, states may waive entry requirements to facilitate both human and animal evacuations and rescues. The State Veterinarian's office or Department of Agriculture can usually provide current information.

## SUMMARY

Keeping people and animals out of harm's way, preventing property loss, and working together in the community with other animal stakeholders and officials are important in building community resilience during disasters. Developing plans for neighbors helping each other evacuate animals is important. Producer helping producer, veterinarian helping veterinarian, and community helping community build resilience by preventing loss, responding to needs, and recovering and restoring livelihoods.

## REFERENCES

1. Heath S, Linnaberry R. Challenges of managing animals in disasters in the U.S. Animals (Basel) 2015;5(2):173–92.
2. California Veterinary Medical Reserve Corps (CAVMRC) Information page. Available at: https://cvma.net/resources/disaster-response-program-2/california-veterinary-medical-reserve-corps-cavmrc/california-veterinary-medical-corps-cavmrc-information/. Accessed January 7, 2018.
3. FEMA emergency support function 11. Available at: https://www.fema.gov/media-library-data/1473679204149-c780047585cbcd6989708920f6b89f15/ESF_11_Ag_and_Natural_Resources_FINAL.pdf. Accessed January 7, 2018.
4. Disaster preparedness for veterinarians. 2018. Available at: https://www.avma.org/kb/resources/reference/disaster/pages/default.aspx. Accessed January 5, 2018.

# Cattle Assessment On-Site During Emergencies

Arthur Lee Jones, DVM, MS[a],*, Renée Dawn Dewell, DVM, MS[b], Joanna Davis, DVM[c]

## KEYWORDS

- Beef cattle • Disaster • Assessment • Veterinary • Emergency

## KEY POINTS

The veterinarian's role and responsibilities may include the following:

- Identification of injured cattle, potential chemical exposure issues, site-specific hazards, and associated potential threats to cattle health and well-being.
- Prioritization of cattle health needs based on clinical observation and/or hands-on assessment of cattle.
- Identification of potential human and animal health hazards and subsequent communication to assessment team members as well as other decision makers.
- Provision of objective and factual information to assist in prevention, treatment, mitigation, and response to diseases affecting beef cattle to responsible regulatory officials or other decision makers.

## INTRODUCTION

A disaster is defined as a sudden calamitous event bringing great damage, loss, or destruction (*Merriam-Webster Dictionary*). Disasters can vary widely in scope, severity, and duration. Disasters may be limited to a sudden, brief event in a limited area or individual farm or encompass large geographic areas such as in a drought. Although natural or weather-related disasters are typically thought of as a disaster, some disasters can be caused directly by human activity, such as toxic spills, arson, or nuclear power plant failures, or exacerbated by human efforts, such as poorly designed flood control levies, dams, or mismanagement of natural resources resulting in catastrophic wildfires. No matter the cause, a disaster creates an emergency: a

Disclosure Statement: The authors have nothing to disclose.
[a] Department of Population Health, TVDIL, UGA College of Veterinary Medicine, PO Box 1389, Tifton, GA 31793, USA; [b] Department of Veterinary Microbiology and Preventive Medicine, Center for Food Security and Public Health, Iowa State University, 1600 South 16th Street, Ames, IA 50011, USA; [c] Emergency Coordinator for Georgia Florida, USDA APHIS Veterinary Services, Surveillance, Preparedness, and Response Services (SPRS), 1506 Klondike Road, Suite 300, Conyers, GA 30094, USA
* Corresponding author.
*E-mail address:* leejones@uga.edu

Vet Clin Food Anim 34 (2018) 233–248
https://doi.org/10.1016/j.cvfa.2018.03.002
0749-0720/18/© 2018 Elsevier Inc. All rights reserved.

situation that presents an immediate risk to health, life, and property requiring immediate action.

Veterinary assessment of the condition and needs of livestock and their owners in an emergency is an essential element of the disaster response. The emergency response for livestock has 4 critical components: assessing the need for and attending to the immediate medical needs of injured or affected livestock, determining the resources available to meet the needs including feed and facilities, identifying any ongoing threats or potential hazards to livestock health and welfare, and appropriate documentation of damages and actions by responders (**Boxes 1** and **2**). Veterinarians may also be asked to communicate findings to owners, agents, or employees associated with the site and the cattle.

This article discusses the veterinarian's role in the assessment of cattle operations during disasters and other types of emergencies. Veterinarians play a key role in the assessment of cattle operations during emergencies and disasters.

In the public health realm, the term "assessment" has been defined as: "The evaluation and interpretation of short and long term measurements to provide a basis for decision making and to enhance public health officials' ability to monitor disaster situations."[1] When this definition is applied to the on-site assessment of beef cattle during emergencies, it may be modified as:

*The evaluation and interpretation of short- and long-term measurements to provide a basis for decision making and to enhance responders' ability to protect, monitor, and improve the health and welfare of beef cattle impacted by natural disasters and other emergencies.*

Human safety must always be prioritized first when undertaking an assessment during an emergency or disaster involving beef cattle. Appropriate planning and preparation are required to successfully conduct assessments. Before performing an assessment, the assessment site should be stable enough to conduct the assessment with minimal risk to human safety. If possible, the assessment team should develop a safety plan and a briefing from a safety officer before beginning the assessment. It is critical that the team clearly understands the goals and mission of the evaluation. The assessment group should prioritize their activities and plans around accomplishing the specific goals of the assessment within the scope of the assignment. The group should understand who to report to, what their defined area of work responsibility is, and what timeframe is required (operations period). For example, if the assignment is to perform a general assessment of conditions and the surrounding environment, then veterinary triage and treatment will be beyond the scope of the work assignment. The assessment group should work within the Incident Command System whenever possible and should clearly understand the chain of command before undertaking the assessment. Observing the chain of command and communication is particularly important when the assessment will occur in austere environments when communication with decision makers may not be reliable. Plans for communication and data collection should account for mobile telephones and other portable technology that may not be functional in the altered environment. Refer to **Box 3** for a suggested list of supplies to procure before arriving at the assessment site. The mission objectives and type of disaster will affect the supplies needed as well as the risks to human safety, training required before assessment, speed of assessment, and protocols.

When conducting cattle operation assessments during emergencies, it is critical to evaluate immediate as well as anticipated needs, available resources, deficiencies, and vulnerabilities of the affected beef cattle population (**Fig. 1**). Information gathered

**Box 1**
**Veterinarians within the DISASTER paradigm**

*Detect*
- Does need exceed resources?
- Extent of damage, how many affected
- Zoonoses surveillance and reporting

*Incident command*
- Operations
- Planning
- Logistics
- Safety

*Scene security and safety*
- Responder safety
- Stability and security of structures where animals are located
- Population/herd health
- Rationing of resources
- Decontamination
- Quarantine-individual versus herd/flock

*Assess hazards*
- Recognition of various pathologic conditions
- Infectious disease prevention and control
- Vector and wildlife control
- Carcass disposal-debris versus public health hazard
- Food and water safety

*Support*
- Preplanning
- Utilization of veterinary schools/clinics to meet surge capacity
- Consider what agencies and organizations may need to assist, make contacts in advance of a disaster
- Licensing and credentialing of volunteers

*Triage and treatment*
- Basic triage
- Consider which wounds, sequelae of each type of disaster
- Determine survivability of animal, humanely euthanize if necessary
- Wound and pain management
- Antibiotic administration, consider withdrawal times
- Mass vaccination and postexposure prophylaxis

*Evacuation*
- Decide early whether farm must evacuate or shelter in place
- Consider feed, water, and shelter/confinement for either scenario
- Long-term management of animals

*Recovery*

- Counseling
- Management of abandoned animals
- Business continuity-market operability, breeding/production cycle disruption
- Insurance and indemnity claims

from on-site cattle assessments during emergencies should be used immediately if the group is planning to assess as well as respond to unmet needs following the evaluation. Alternatively, the assessment may be used by decision makers or field-level responders to take action based on the gathered information and subsequent identified needs.

To obtain data concerning cattle health needs, assessments are conducted on-site using data gathered from key people, such as cattle owners, managers, extension agents, and other relevant sources. Safety concerns may prevent cattle owners from being present on-site during the assessment. If one or more key people are not present during the assessment, an interview should be arranged before the assessment to gather preliminary data as well as after the assessment to help fill in data gaps when possible. Data are also gathered by walking or driving around the site and by directly observing the cattle on-site whenever possible. Depending on the type and scope of the emergency or disaster as well as the hazards associated with the physical environment, animals in unfamiliar surroundings may be nervous, panicked, and confused and may not behave normally.[2]

A primary role of a veterinarian conducting beef cattle assessments during emergencies is to prioritize cattle health needs based on assessment of the physical environment, animal husbandry needs, and clinical observation and/or physical examination of cattle. A rapid response to urgent needs should not be delayed because a comprehensive assessment has not yet been completed. Available resources, gaps, and vulnerabilities for the affected beef cattle population should be identified for both long- and short-term action. Information gathered from on-site cattle assessments during emergencies can be used immediately if the group is planning to assess as well as respond to unmet needs following the evaluation.

Critical needs for cattle typically include access to clean water and food and intact, proper fencing. After an emergency, existing site infrastructure may be damaged, inoperable, inaccessible, or otherwise unusable. It may be necessary to evaluate cattle health and well-being from a distance without the use of cattle handling equipment, such as chutes or small pens. Veterinarians may benefit from the use of binoculars to evaluate cattle populations. In some cases, aerial assessments of cattle operations may be preferred.

An assessment that takes place shortly after a disaster or emergency occurs is sometimes referred to as a "rapid needs assessment," or RNA,[3] or an initial rapid assessment (IRA).[4] An RNA/IRA is meant to adopt a population-based approach to assessment, which lends itself well to production animal medicine. Information obtained from an RNA/INA is used to determine gaps, define tangible and intangible resources that are needed, and address the most immediate needs of the beef cattle population being evaluated. Inspectors should also be able to determine whether additional resources will be needed after taking care of the most pressing needs.

**Box 2**
**Suggested inventory and supplies for livestock evacuation kit**

- 10- to 14-day supply of feed, hay, supplements, and potable water supply
- Feed buckets
- Livestock marking crayon, nontoxic, non-water-soluble spray paint, or markers to write on the animal's side
- Batteries (flashlight, radio), chargers (including solar powered)
- Boots/appropriate footwear, N95 disposable face masks
- Blankets
- Copies of veterinary and other medical records
- Proof of ownership for each animal and piece of equipment
- Cotton or leather halters
- Duct tape
- Emergency contact list
- First aid kit (see item suggestions in the "Saving the Whole Family" brochure)
- Flashlight
- Fly spray
- Heavy gloves (leather)
- Hoof nippers
- Instructions
  - Any special handling or management guidelines
  - Medications: list each animal separately, and for each medication include the drug name, dosage, and frequency (include treatment start date and withdrawal times)
- Knife (sharp, all-purpose)
- Paper maps of local area and alternate evacuation routes in addition to GPS (in case of road closures)
- Paper towels, trash bags, disinfectant
- Plastic trash cans with lids (can be used to store water)
- Portable livestock panels and/or rolls of polypropylene snow fencing, stakes for fencing
- Radio (solar, hand cranked, and/or battery operated)
- Ropes or lariat, carbingers of different sizes
- Shovel, hammer
- Tarpaulins
- Water buckets
- Wire cutters
- Waste management equipment
- Clippers/shearers
- Nose tongs
- Spray paint, sharpies
- Generators
- Backup communications such as 2-way radio

*Adapted from* AVMA's "Saving the Whole Family." Available at: www.avma.org/disaster; with permission. Accessed November 23, 2017.

---

**Box 3**
**Example of supplies that may be useful to bring to a beef cattle operation assessment**

Coveralls

Gloves (leather/canvass and/or surgical)

Writing tools that write on wet paper

Assessment paperwork

Ropes

Euthanasia supplies

Flashlight

Communications device

Hardhat

Boots (steel toed or otherwise appropriate)

Disinfecting supplies

Clipboard

Camera

Dart gun

Necropsy supplies

First aid kit

Safety glasses

Ziploc bags (for electronics and paperwork)

---

The World Health Organization developed an IRA form with 6 sections,[4] which may be modified as listed below for beef cattle assessment in an emergency:

- Beef cattle population description
- Shelter, fencing, facilities
- Available potable water supply
- Forage/ration security, including condition and availability
- Cattle health status and current or potential health risks
- Potential zoonoses

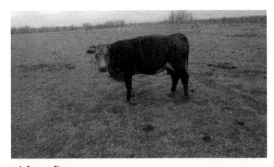

**Fig. 1.** A cow injured from fire.

## BEEF CATTLE POPULATION DESCRIPTION

The number and class of cattle on-site should be estimated or determined from available records at the onset of the assessment. A brief population description should also be included in the assessment. The type of production enterprises, such as cow-calf, feedlot, or stocker/backgrounder, should be noted. General demeanor and disposition of the herd should also be noted. If present, bulls should be included in the description, and other assessment team members should be made aware of the bull's presence.

## SHELTER, FENCING, FACILITIES

Beef cattle are often sheltered in place, although they may become displaced from their premises as a result of the disaster. If fencing exists, it should be checked for structural soundness and safety. Depending on the type of disaster or emergency, flying objects may have been tossed into areas that cattle inhabit. The area the cattle are residing in should be checked for potential hazards that may have made their way into their pasture or pen. Identify any animals that may have been injured by debris or projectiles. If possible, hazards associated with debris that pose an imminent threat to cattle health and safety should be mitigated during the assessment by moving or covering them. Facilities and grounds should also be checked for signs of potential chemical releases, the security of farm chemicals, and downed electrical lines noted. Electricity to power boxes should be turned to the off position and not turned back on until inspected by an electrician.

The footing should also be evaluated. If possible, cattle should have access to a dry area to stand or lay. If there are no dry areas in the enclosures or pasture and heavy equipment is available, it may be possible to recommend that operators build a mound that cattle can access for a dry area for resting and feeding.

If there are working facilities, such as small pens, alleys, tubs, and chutes, they should be noted on the assessment. A cursory evaluation of their fitness for use should be completed and noted on the assessment. A determination of existing facilities and equipment should be made regarding the fitness of facilities to evaluate cattle in small groups or individually.

## AVAILABLE WATER SUPPLY

In many cases, adequate amounts of clean water may be the most limited resource. When assessing existing or needed resources for affected cattle, identification of a safe water source is the most immediate nutritional need. Generators may be needed to pump water from a well if the electricity is out for a prolonged period. Chemicals, sewage, or carcasses may be a potential source of water contamination following a disaster.

## FORAGE/RATION SECURITY

Availability and access to an adequate amount of unspoiled hay or other forage are important to verify during an assessment. Stored forage and grain sources should be evaluated for dryness and for evidence of spoilage or contaminants. If cattle are on pasture, the pasture should be checked for evidence of damage due to the disaster, presence of debris, overgrazing, and the presence of toxic plants. If pastures in coastal areas are flooded with saltwater, grasses may die quickly, leaving animals without forage. If adequate forage is not available, cattle may graze the toxic plants, and this possible hazard should be noted in the assessment. Based on the population type, number, and production phase and type, an estimate should be made regarding the length of time any available stored forages and grains as well natural forages should be available for cattle. If adequate feed is not available, this should be noted on the assessment. Depending on the type of disaster or emergency, high-quality feedstuffs may be limited. In this case, lesser-quality feedstuffs may be substituted as needed to sustain adequate body condition. If appropriate and adequate feed is not available and cannot be procured in a timely manner, euthanasia or transportation should be considered for humane reasons. Please see J.W. Waggoner and K.C. Olson's article, "Feeding and Watering Beef Cattle During Disasters," in this issue, for additional guidance regarding feedstuffs during an emergency or disaster.

## CATTLE HEALTH STATUS AND CURRENT OR POTENTIAL RISKS

During the initial on-site assessment, the magnitude and extent of the emergency should be determined. The assessor may observe the herd to determine the estimated:

- Number of cattle on-site
- Production type and stage
- Ownership of cattle on-site, identification and/or brands (do they belong on the premises or have they been displaced from another premises?)
- Hydration status
- Body condition scores
- Morbidities other than traumatic injury
- Mortalities
- Types of injuries
- Temperament and disposition
- Presence and type of other species

If possible, owners or managers of the cattle being evaluated should be consulted regarding the overall health of their cattle and any special or ongoing needs, recent health problems, or if the cattle are being treated for disease, for injury, or with medications. If treatment records are available, they should be consulted, and recently treated animals should be visually evaluated. Special attention should be given to the most vulnerable populations, such as younger calves, pregnant females, and special-needs cattle in treatment or sick pens. Compared with other cattle on-site, these populations may require maintenance on a higher level of nutrition, access to shelter, and more intensive medical attention.

When assessing cow-calf pairs, it is important to allow the pairs to "mother up" so that it is clear that each suckling calf has a live dam associated with it. If there are mortalities or morbidities involving cows, attempt to identify the corresponding calf. If the sick or dead cow is part of a pair and the calf is too young to be weaned, then alternative means to care for the calf will need to be identified and readily implemented.

## VETERINARY TRIAGE

Although environmental disasters do not typically result in veterinary emergencies among cattle, morbidities and mortalities do occur.[5] Similarly, some types of environmental disasters as well as other types of emergencies may necessitate veterinary triage. Veterinary triage is conducted with the "purpose of doing the greatest good for the largest number of animals."[6] It balances the veterinary medical needs of the individual animal with the available veterinary resources.

It is important to recognize that time and resources are often limited. Thus, normal treatment protocols may not be used in these circumstances. Animals that are most likely to benefit from available care should be the most likely to be treated. In contrast to triage systems in human disaster medicine, veterinary medicine has the option of euthanasia (please see Jan K. Shearer and colleagues' article, "Humane Euthanasia and Carcass Disposal," in this issue) (**Fig. 2**). Veterinary triage for emergencies involving beef cattle will likely have little tolerance for outcomes that will negatively impact long-term health and production performance or potentially pose a food safety hazard. Triage decisions may also be affected by the following:

- Available veterinary personnel
- Available veterinary medical equipment and supplies
- Number of affected animals and amount of time required to alleviate the condition
- Required follow-up care
- Stability or availability of needed infrastructure, such as fencing or shelter
- Available transportation and/or road conditions
- Access to feed and potable water
- Production phase or genetic value
- Temperament of the animal
- Estimated value of animal
- Emotional attachment of owner
- Likelihood of presumed diagnosis to be transmitted to other animals or to people

Cattle will likely be assessed in a field situation, and the assessing veterinarian should be prepared to triage animals into categories based on observation and assessment in the field. Animals should be observed for the following:

- Ability to ambulate normally
- Body condition score
- Evidence of trauma
- Evidence of other diseases, such as respiratory disease, or chemical contamination, including ingestion

If animals are identified with abnormal ambulation (lameness), a scoring system may be helpful to evaluate and record their locomotion (**Table 1**).

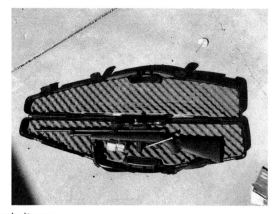

**Fig. 2.** A dart gun in its case.

**Table 1**
Locomotion scoring for beef cattle

| | Locomotion and Mobility Numerical Score Category | | | | | |
| | Finished Cattle Locomotion Scoring Systems | | | | | |
| | 0 | 1 | 2 | 3 | 4 | 5 |
|---|---|---|---|---|---|---|
| NAMI Mobility Scoring System[11] | | Normal: walks easily with no apparent lameness or change in gait | Exhibits minor stiffness, shortness of stride, or a slight limp but keeps up with normal cattle in the group | Exhibits obvious stiffness, difficulty taking steps, an obvious limp or obvious discomfort, and lags behind normal cattle walking as a group | Extremely reluctant to move even when encouraged by a handler; described as statuelike | |
| Terrell,[12] 2016 | Normal: animal walks normally; no apparent lameness or change in gait | Mild lameness: animal exhibits shortened stride, may move head slightly side to side but no head bob | Moderate lameness: animal exhibits a limp, with an obviously identifiable limb or limbs affected and/or head bob present when walking; limbs still bear weight | Severe lameness: animal applies little or no weight to affected limb while standing or walking; animal reluctant or unable to move. Although walking, animal's head dropped, back arched, with head bob and limp detected | | |
| Step-Up Locomotion Scoring System[13] | Normal: animal walks normally with no apparent lameness or change in gait; hind feet land in a similar location to front feet | Mild lameness: animal exhibits short stride when walking, dropping its head slightly; animal does not exhibit a limp when walking | Moderate lameness: animal exhibits obvious limp, favoring affected limbs, which still bear weight; a slight head bob is present when the animal is walking | Severe lameness: animal applies little or no weight to affected limb and is reluctant or unable to move. Although walking, animal's head is dropped and back arched, with head bob and limp detected | | |

From Edwards-Callaway LN, Calvo-Lorenzo MS, Scanga JA, et al. Mobility scoring of finished cattle. Vet Clin North Am Food Anim Pract 2017;33(2):238-9; with permission.

Animals that show the following conditions should be identified as potentially compromised. If possible, and within the scope of the assessment mission, they should be individually examined for further triage:

- Moribund
- Nonambulatory
- Severely lame
- Have a body condition score of less than 2 on a scale of 1 to 9[7]
- Show signs of being visually impaired
- Have evidence of severe trauma
- Show signs of other diseases

If animals have been exposed to flood waters or other potential toxicants, it is important to grossly decontaminate them before individual examination. If a gross decontamination is not immediately possible, veterinarians and others that may have direct contact with the animal should be trained in the effective use of personal protective equipment (PPE) and wear appropriate PPE to protect themselves from exposure to potential hazards. After individual examination of compromised animals and depending on the available resources and scope of the mission, compromised animals may be treated or humanely euthanized. If euthanasia activities are conducted, it is important to consider the emotional impact of euthanasia on the owner.

## POTENTIAL ZOONOSES

It is a commonly held belief that there is an increased risk of communicable or zoonotic diseases following a disaster, particularly a flood affecting a large geographic region. However, there is little scientific evidence that supports a link of natural disasters to significant and consistent increases in the incidence of infectious diseases of animals.[8] The actual risk factors for outbreaks threatening to human and livestock health are displacement of animals and potentially people, lack of adequate veterinary care, lack of clean water and adequate feed, crowded conditions, poor sanitation,[9] and increased exposure to wildlife that may be displaced during a disaster.[8]

Increased incidence of infectious disease outbreaks caused by leptospirosis, cryptosporidiosis, giardiasis, mosquito-borne diseases, and anthrax has been cited as concerns due to water contaminated with these or other organisms.[8] Flooding may also contribute to an uptick in mosquito populations, but many of the mosquito species are nuisance species and not vectors for transmitting diseases.[8] Precious resources may be exhausted attempting to prevent zoonotic outbreaks that are not likely to occur anyway. Animal health professionals may be better advised to address the known environmental risk factors that contribute to disease following a disaster, stabilize the environment, provide proper care for animals, and implement appropriate prophylactic measures to control known risks of disease transmission.

### Disaster Mitigation on Farms

The most effective disaster response begins with thorough planning and preparation to mitigate its impact. Studies have shown that for every $1 invested in risk reduction (mitigation), communities save an average of $4 in resource costs.[10] Most importantly, disaster planning and preparations save lives of both animals and humans. Just as producers plan the herd's breeding, nutrition, disease and parasite control, so too should they invest in protecting their animals from the impacts of disasters. In an instant, one's economic investment, animal genetics, and way of life may be obliterated, but veterinarians can work with producers to minimize the impact of a catastrophe. Developing an emergency response plan before a disaster can reduce the loss of life, property, and businesses, prioritize needs, improve communication during an event, foster partnership development, and save producers' and taxpayers' money.

Although all risks cannot be completely eliminated, there are practical steps veterinarians and producers can take to mitigate the negative outcomes of a disaster. On a national scale, Federal Emergency Management Agency (FEMA) has published the National Preparedness Goal that offers guidance to communities and states on how to prevent, protect, mitigate, respond to, and recover from a variety of disasters and emergencies, including terrorism. These 5 mission areas offer a simple outline for how one can begin to build a disaster preparedness plan. Begin by identifying the major disaster risk factors in the area. Once major vulnerabilities have been identified, a series of "what if" questions should be asked to address concerns.

Families should have their own personal preparedness and response plan to protect their lives, and producers may use the resources available to plan for their operations. For example, would a producer be able to evacuate animals, or do they have a means to care for them if they cannot be evacuated? All animals should have permanent identification, and the producer should keep current records of animal identification so stray animals can be returned. Microchips and brands are ideal because ear tags may get torn or burned out of an ear, or may be so dirty they are illegible. If possible, producers should take individual photographs of all animals, including a close-up of their head and a side view or any distinguishing marks. A photograph of the animal may be valuable if animals become displaced, or for documenting animal inventory for insurance or disaster relief claims.

In recent disasters, availability and accessibility of feed and potable water have been an issue. Investing in backup generators in the event of prolonged power outages may help provide water from well pumps that operate with electricity. During a disaster, it may be difficult to purchase generators because the rest of the community may be impacted. Consider fuel storage options during a disaster for vehicles, generators, and other farm equipment. Cell towers and telephone lines may be damaged in a disaster, and producers should consider alternative methods of communication, such as satellite telephones, ham radios, and 2-way radios. **Box 3** provides an inventory and supply list.

### Develop Partnerships Before a Disaster

Producers should make a plan for who is responsible for what activities in case of evacuation. Determine who will gather animals and where, who will transport the animals, who will gather feed and other supplies, and what route the driver will take, and where everyone will meet. If not evacuating animals, decide who will care for animals. Producers can work with neighbors to make a specific plan now about how they may respond alongside each other, sharing resources and caring for animals.

Veterinarians and producers should meet and work with county emergency managers and other first responders before a disaster strikes. They may help producers in the planning process during "peacetime" and are an invaluable resource during an emergency. It is beneficial for the County Emergency Management Agency to be aware of where the farm is located, how many animals are at each location, and what kind of structures and utilities are on the property. It may also be beneficial to take free online introductory courses on emergency management offered by FEMA (see links in the appendix). Governmental emergency response agencies function under the Incident Command System, and the courses address basic emergency response language, organization, and response and may provide credentialing for county response volunteers.

Extension agents are also very important team members and can work with multiple farms in the area to develop a countywide plan, including the identification of shelters accepting large animals, pets, and available resources in the area and may assist in the response and recovery efforts. The Farm Service Agency and Small Business Administration both offer disaster relief loans or reimbursement for losses. Producers and veterinarians can familiarize themselves with the information or documentation these or other agencies may require for citizens seeking relief following a disaster. See the Appendix for links to these agencies and the disaster aid each may offer. It is important to submit accurate documentation soon after a disaster because most loans are considered on a first-come, first-served basis. Keep in mind that these loans will not provide immediate relief. It is vital that producers have adequate cash or immediate access to other funds the first several weeks after a disaster. Banks may be closed, ATMs may not work, and businesses may not extend credit after a disaster. If animals died or their breeding cycle was interrupted by the effects of a disaster, consider how to replace the income the farm may lose during the downtime, and how the farm will be restocked. Depending on the extent of the disaster, local markets and slaughterhouses may not be operational as an option for disposition of animals.

### Governmental Response to Disasters

It is important to remember that *all* disaster response begins locally. Some state or federal resources may be staged when a disaster such as a hurricane can be predicted, but local/county resources will respond initially. When local resources have been exhausted (or are expected to be), local governments may request a gubernatorial disaster declaration to provide state level resources to a disaster response. If the state resources are (or expected to be) exhausted, a Governor may request a federal disaster declaration to provide federal resources for a catastrophic disaster. Each level of government must request assistance from the next highest level for assistance; the state or federal government may not respond without the request. It could take days or weeks to mobilize all requested resources to a disaster-affected area. It is imperative that a farm is prepared to be self-sustaining in austere conditions in a major disaster. Government resources may be limited, and responders may not be able to safely reach one's property for several days after a disaster.

As a farm and community begin rebuilding after the disaster, consider what could be done differently to mitigate the impacts of disaster next time. What lessons were learned and what improvements could be made in preparation for the next disaster? It is important to be a leader before the next emergency, to devise a plan *and* a backup plan to respond when communities are impacted by a disaster.

### REFERENCES

1. Landesman LY. Appendix A. In: Public health management of disasters: the practical guide. Washington, DC: The American Public Health Association; 2001. p. 169.
2. Cotton S, McBride T. Caring for livestock during disaster. Colorado State University Extension: Livestock Series Management; 2013. Available at: http://extension.colostate.edu/docs/pubs/livestk/01815.pdf. Accessed November 11, 2017.

3. Cranmer HH, McKay MP. Rapid needs assessments. In: Kapur GB, Smith JP, editors. Emergency public health preparedness and response. Sudbury (Canada): Jones and Bartlett Learning; 2011. p. 185–98.

4. World Health Organization. Initial rapid assessment (IRA): field assessment form. 2009. Available at: http://www.who.int/hac/network/global_health_cluster/ira_form_v2_7_eng.pdf. Accessed November 11, 2017.

5. Shearer J, Irsik M, Zimmel D, et al. Livestock and horses: emergency management for large animals. 2007. Available at: http://www.flsart.org/pdf/LAH-EMG-LP-2007-06.pdf. Accessed November 11, 2017.

6. Wingfield WE. Section 1.9 veterinary triage. In: Wingfield WE, Palmer SB, editors. Veterinary disaster response. Ames (IA): Wiley-Blackwell; 2009. p. 111–21. Philadelphia: 2017. p. 235–50.

7. Stewart L, Dyer T. Body condition scoring beef cows. Available at: http://www.cowbcs.info/pdf/BCS_Update.pdf. Accessed November 11, 2017.

8. Animal health hazards of concern during natural disasters. United States Department of Agriculture Animal and Plant Health Inspection Service Veterinary Services; 2002. Available at: https://www.aphis.usda.gov/animal_health/emergingissues/downloads/hazards.PDF. Accessed November 28, 2017.

9. Watson JT, Gayer M, Connolly MA. Epidemics after natural disasters. Emerg Infect Dis 2007;13(1):1.

10. Godschalk DR, Rose A, Mittler E, et al. Estimating the value of foresight: aggregate analysis of natural hazard mitigation benefits and costs. J Environ Plann Manag 2009;52(6):739–56.

11. NAMI. North American Meat Institute Mobility Scoring System 2016. Available at: https://www.youtube.com/watch?v=QIslfHCvkpg. Accessed April 2, 2018.

12. Terrell SP. Feedlot lameness: industry perceptions, locomotion scoring, lameness morbidity, and association of locomotion score and diagnosis with case outcome in beef cattle in Great Plains feedlots. Manhattan (KS): Kansas State University; 2016.

13. Step-Up® Locomotion Scoring System. Zinpro Corporation 2016. Available at: http://www.zinpro.com/lameness/beef/locomotion-scoring. Accessed April 2, 2018.

## APPENDIX 1

*Resources*

*Veterinary Disasters & Emergencies*
**Training:** ***Please keep copies of all of your certificates of completion for any courses that you take. For involvement in local, county, or state teams, you may need to show proof of training to be able to participate.***

- ICS 100-Introduction to the Incident Command System, (free training) http://training.fema.gov/is/courseoverview.aspx?code=IS-100.b
- ICS 200-Enables personnel to operate efficiently during an incident or event within the Incident Command System (free training) http://www.training.fema.gov/is/courseoverview.aspx?code=IS-200.b
- ICS 700-introduces and overviews the National Incident Management System (NIMS), a nationwide template to enable all government, private-sector, and nongovernmental organizations to work together during domestic incidents. https://training.fema.gov/is/courseoverview.aspx?code=IS-700.a

IS 10A-Animals in Disasters: Awareness and Preparedness (free training) http://www.training.fema.gov/is/courseoverview.aspx?code=IS-10.a

IS 11-Animals in Disasters, Module B: Community Planning (free training) http://www.training.fema.gov/is/courseoverview.aspx?code=IS-11.a

IS 111-Livestock in Disasters (free training) http://www.training.fema.gov/is/courseoverview.aspx?code=IS-111.a

Video-properly donning and doffing Personal Protective Equipment (PPE) http://www.usdatraining.com/ppe/

Ready AG© Workbook from Penn State Extension (PDF) is designed to help farm and ranch owners be better prepared to deal with disasters that can occur on their farm or ranch such as power outages, drought, flood, severe snow- or ice storms, including catastrophic events as tornadoes, hurricanes, fires, disease outbreaks, and acts of terrorism or a nuclear accident. Filled with checklists, worksheets, and map templates for producers to complete before a disaster. https://extension.psu.edu/readyag-workbook

American Veterinary Medical Association (AVMA) Disaster Preparedness information for veterinarians and clients www.avma.org/disaster

AVMA Disaster Reimbursement Grants-Up to $5,000 may be issued per grantee for out-of-pocket expenses incurred by veterinarians providing emergency veterinary medical care to animal victims of disasters. Issued on first come, first served basis as long as funds are available. https://www.avmf.org/for-veterinarians/disaster-reimbursement-grants/

Iowa State University Center for Food Security & Public Health-Resources on zoonotic diseases, emergency management, business continuity management, free online courses, agroterror, educational opportunities www.cfsph.iastate.edu

FEMA National Preparedness Goal- describes methods for the whole community to prevent, protect against, mitigate, respond to, and recover from the threats and hazards that pose the greatest risk. https://www.fema.gov/national-preparedness-goal

FEMA Business Continuity planning- www.ready.gov/business/index.html

Small Business Administration Disaster Loans-Low interest loans for homeowner, businesses and renters affected by declared disasters. https://www.sba.gov/funding-programs/disaster-assistance

Technical Large Animal Emergency Rescue- www.tlaer.org the practical Considerations, Behavioral Understanding, Specialty Equipment, Techniques, Methodologies and Tactics behind the safe extrication of a live large animal from entrapments (trailer wrecks, ditches, mud, barn fires) in local emergencies and disaster areas.

Farm MAPPER -This project explores using Quick Response tags (QR codes) to provide emergency responders on-site information about hazards and physical layouts of agricultural operations. http://www.nfmcfarmmapper.com/Home/About

Ranch Aid- RanchAid provides a framework for coordination and cooperation across Private, Government, and Non-Government organizations (NGO) regarding agricultural animal incidents affecting the health, safety, and welfare of communities and animals. www.ranchaid.org

Code 3 Associates- Provides professional animal disaster response and resources to communities, as well as providing professional training to individuals and agencies involved in animal related law enforcement and emergency response through hands-on animal rescue and care operations during disaster events in the United States and Canada. http://code3associates.org/

*Farm Service Agency (FSA) Disaster Assistance Programs:*
It is recommended to review these programs during *preparations* so that producers may maintain appropriate documentation in case of a disaster. There are submission deadlines, and requests are considered on a first come, first served basis.

- https://www.fsa.usda.gov/programs-and-services/disaster-assistance-program/index
- Livestock Indemnity Program (LIP) factsheet- LIP provides benefits to livestock producers for livestock deaths in excess of normal mortality caused by adverse weather or by attacks by animals reintroduced into the wild by the federal government
- https://www.fsa.usda.gov/Assets/USDA-FSA-Public/usdafiles/FactSheets/2017/lip_fact_sheet_oct2017.pdf
- Livestock Forage Program (LFP): LFP provides compensation to eligible livestock producers that have suffered grazing losses due to drought or fire on land that is native or improved pastureland with permanent vegetative cover or that is planted specifically for grazing.
- https://www.fsa.usda.gov/Assets/USDA-FSA-Public/usdafiles/FactSheets/2017/livestock_forage_disaster_program_oct2017.pdf
- Emergency Assistance for Livestock, Honeybees, and Farm-Raised Fish (ELAP): ELAP provides emergency assistance to eligible producers of livestock, honeybees and farm-raised fish for losses due to disease (including cattle tick fever), adverse weather, or other conditions, such as blizzards and wildfires, not covered by LFP and LIP.
- https://www.fsa.usda.gov/Assets/USDA-FSA-Public/usdafiles/FactSheets/2017/elap_for_livestock_oct2017.pdf
- Check with state departments of agriculture, state animal health officials/state veterinarians, and state veterinary medical associations for other information on preparedness and response in your state.

# Feeding and Watering Beef Cattle During Disasters

Justin W. Waggoner, MS, PhD[a],*, K.C. Olson, MS, PhD[b]

## KEYWORDS

• Emergency • Disaster • Nutrition • Cattle • Management

## KEY POINTS

• Emergency nutrition and management of cattle comprise 2 phases: survival and maintenance.
• The basic elements of feeding and management essential for survival of cattle following a natural disaster are water, feed, rest, and recovery.
• The secondary objective is to maintain the current condition of cattle and reduce the potential for negative production outcomes.
• General recommendations for both survival and maintenance following natural disasters, including flooding, blizzards, and wildfire, are discussed.

## INTRODUCTION

The objective of this article is to provide a general overview of feeding, watering, and managing beef cattle following select natural disasters or emergency situations. The authors rely primarily on personal experience in relating successes and failures in managing livestock-related emergencies; however, the experiences and research of others are cited when appropriate.

No 2 natural disasters or emergencies that impact livestock are alike, and each situation will have unique challenges. Animal care, feeding, and nutrition in the wake of a natural disaster or emergency require a general understanding of animal nutrient requirements, feedstuffs, creativity, and perseverance.

## EMERGENCY PREPAREDNESS AND MANAGING DONATED FEEDSTUFFS

One the most challenging aspects of feeding and caring for livestock in emergency situations is the logistics associated with the management and allocation of donated feedstuffs. Incident-response personnel should identify a central person of contact

Disclosure Statement: The authors have nothing to disclose.
[a] Southwest Research and Extension Center, Kansas State University, 4500 East Mary Street, Garden City, KS 67846, USA; [b] Department of Animal Sciences and Industry, Kansas State University, 126 Call Hall, Manhattan, KS 66506, USA
* Corresponding author.
E-mail address: jwaggon@ksu.edu

Vet Clin Food Anim 34 (2018) 249–257
https://doi.org/10.1016/j.cvfa.2018.02.006
0749-0720/18/Published by Elsevier Inc.

vetfood.theclinics.com

that has some knowledge of feedstuffs, animal needs, and livestock producers in the area. A location for use as a receiving point and staging area for donated feeds should also be identified as soon as possible after the event. The staging area should be large enough to accommodate large volumes of hay and have covered storage available to accommodate bagged feeds or concentrates. The staging area should be accessible also from major roadways; it should be marked with obvious signage, and it should have available the heavy equipment necessary to handle various types of feeds on hand. An effort should be made to allocate and direct feedstuffs directly to producers, when possible, to ease pressure and space constraints at the staging area. Although difficult, the name and location of the feedstuff donor, any pertinent information regarding the donated feedstuffs (eg, identity, nutrient analysis, and nitrate content), and the name and location of the recipient of donated feedstuffs should be documented. If any problems (ie, toxicities, contamination, or presence of noxious or invasive forage species) with specific feeds become known at a later date, the recipients of those feeds can be notified immediately so that steps to mitigate unintended consequences can be taken. Donated feeds will vary considerably in terms of type, form, quality, and nutrient composition. Incoming feedstuffs should be allocated based on the relative nutrient requirements of animals being cared for and the resources available to the recipient to handle and store different types of feedstuffs. Producers should be put into contact with University Extension professionals, nutritionists, or veterinarians to seek advice regarding the use of unfamiliar feedstuffs or feeds that may have unique characteristics (ie, heat damage). Donated hay should also be monitored for contaminants (ie, foreign objects) that may injure animals or damage hay-processing equipment.

## GENERAL WATER AND FEEDING MANAGEMENT CONSIDERATIONS

Maintaining cattle on limited resources for any duration of time is inherently difficult and requires skillful management. Immediately following a natural disaster (ie, 2–3 days; the survival phase), the most basic needs for survival of cattle (ie, water, feed, rest, and recovery) are of primary importance. Once the survival phase has been addressed, the secondary objective is to maintain the present condition of cattle (ie, the maintenance phase) and to reduce the potential for negative production outcomes, such as severe body weight loss or pregnancy loss.

### Survival Phase

---

**Key survival phase considerations**

*Water (First priority)*
- 1.0 to 2.0 gallons per 100 lbs body weight
- Introduce slowly if cattle have been without access for >12 hours
- Provide tank space for 10% of animals, allowing 1 linear foot of tank space per head

*Feed (second priority)*
- Offer 1.0% to 1.5% body weight per day of long-stemmed moderate-quality forage (grass hay preferred)
- Restrict grain and other supplements to 0.5% body weight per day
- Limit intake of unfamiliar feeds

- Cattle should have access to abundant, clean drinking water. The amount of water required varies. In general, cattle will consume approximately 1.0 to 2.0 gallons of water per 100 lbs of body weight. Water availability may need to be increased slowly if cattle have not had access to water for periods in excess of 12 hours.[1] Keep in mind that water requirements may vary greatly with ambient temperature, relative humidity, animal health status, and existence of physical trauma.[2] Water consumption may range from 300% to 800% of dry matter intake in terms of water weight. Take care also to provide adequate access to water-delivery vessels for cattle in confinement. The following rules of thumb and calculations may be useful when estimating the number and size of water tanks needed for a given situation:
  - Provide drinking access = 10% of total animals in enclosure 1 linear foot per head
  - 1 gallon of water = 8.3 lbs
  - 1 cubic foot of water = 7.48 gallons or 62.3 pounds
  - 1 gallon or water = 231 cubic inches

$$\text{Circular trough capacity, gallons} = \frac{3.14 \times \text{radius}^2 \times \text{depth (in inches)}}{231}$$

$$\text{Rectangular trough capacity, gallons} = \frac{\text{length} \times \text{width} \times \text{height (in inches)}}{231}$$

Gallons by inch of depth = total gallons ÷ tank depth, inches

- Feed intake of cattle immediately following a disaster will often be low because of the stress associated with the event. Therefore, initially offering cattle 1% to 1.5% of their body weight of palatable, long-stemmed moderate-quality forage (grass hay, if possible) should satiate the animals and reduce waste of feed resources that, in some cases, may be limited. Concentrate feedstuffs should be restricted to 0.5% of body weight.
- Abrupt diet transitions should be addressed within the first 3 days following the traumatic event by either limiting intake of unfamiliar feeds or offering feedstuffs that have a similar nutrient composition and profile to those the cattle were fed before the event.
- Cattle should be allowed to rest, if possible, before trucking or imposing additional stressors, such as sorting, commingling, or processing.

### Maintenance Phase

- The most vulnerable cattle at risk for production losses in an emergency situation are animals with the highest nutrient requirements: newborn calves, lactating females, and pregnant females. Cattle should be sorted into management groups based on stage of production and nutrient requirements if possible. Sorting cattle into groups based on stage of production facilitates more accurate delivery of feedstuffs and reduces the likelihood of underfeeding specific classes of cattle and maximizes use of resources.
- The most critical elements of cattle nutrition in an emergency situation are energy, protein, and macrominerals (ie, calcium, phosphorous, potassium, and sodium). This does not diminish the importance or essentiality of other

macrominerals or microminerals in the diets of beef cattle; however, the afore-mentioned mineral elements are those upon which a primary emphasis should be placed in an emergency situation. They are the most rapidly depleted during times of injury, dehydration, starvation, or other stress and are vital for restoring normal electrolyte balance.

- The maintenance energy requirements of nonlactating pregnant beef cows, mature bulls, and weaned calves in most cases can be met with moderate-quality forages (6%–12% crude protein, 50% total digestible nutrients, dry matter basis) at an expected daily dry matter intake of approximately 2.0% to 2.5% body weight. Grass hays are often recommended for stressed cattle. However, grass hays and forages in general are frequently protein poor; there-fore, additional supplemental protein is often warranted. Feeding a minimum of 1 lb per day of a 20% to 30% crude protein supplement will supply additional nitrogen to the rumen and improve forage digestion and utilization. Protein sup-plements include, but are not limited to, oilseed meals, corn gluten feed, dried distillers grain, and legume hays.

- Cattle should be fed daily, and no more than a 1- to 2-day supply of hay should be offered at any one time. This amount of hay will minimize wastage of poten-tially limited feed resources and reduce pressure on grazed forage resources of limited availability.

- Combination supplements that provide both energy and protein are ideal in emergency situations, because both may be limited.

- In emergency situations hay may not be immediately available or it may be impractical to or impossible to transport large amounts of hay. In these circum-stances, feeding limited amounts of fiber-based concentrates or grains (eg, dried distiller's grains, corn gluten feed, or soybean hulls) or limited amounts of starch-based concentrates (eg, corn, sorghum, barley, or wheat) may be considered a means of maintaining cattle, when grazed or harvested forage supplies are limited.[3] Initially, care should be taken to limit intake of starch-based concentrates to no more than 0.5% of animal body weight, especially when animals have had no or limited access to such feedstuffs previously. Intake of starch-based concentrates sources can be safely increased 0.5 to 1 lb per adult animal every 2 to 4 days, provided a reasonable forage allowance is also maintained.

- Feed exogenous sources of hay (ie, donations from outside of a disaster-stricken area) in locations that can be monitored in subsequent growing seasons for the presence of noxious plant species.

## EMERGENCY FEEDING DURING FLOODS

The primary concern for livestock owners following regional flooding is usually quality of available water and feed. Flood conditions, in general, may contaminate livestock water in 1 of 2 ways. In inland areas, shallow wells and surface-water sources (ie, ponds) may become contaminated with debris, farm chemicals, petroleum products, decaying organic matter, or sewage after a flood. Each affected water source must be evaluated on a case-by-case basis. Water should only be considered clean after comprehensive testing for mineral content (including heavy metals), coliforms, and hy-drocarbons confirms its safety. In circumstances whereby a visual inspection reveals obvious contamination, use of affected water sources must be avoided until decon-tamination can be achieved. When contamination is less obvious, water sources can be evaluated by sight, feel, or smell for the presence of suspicious odors, pigments, or oily residues. In dire emergencies and for short periods of time, contaminated water that does not contain oily residues may be cleaned using unscented chlorine bleach. In the case of surface water, 1 to 2 gallons of chlorine bleach (5.25% strength) will treat 100 gallons of water. In the case of a shallow well, a solution consisting of 1 gallon of unscented chlorine bleach and 3 gallons of water can be poured into the well bore. Hydrants or faucets that are fed by the well should be opened until the odor of bleach is detected; once this occurs, all hydrant and faucet valves should be shut. After a 24-hour wait, the well should be safe to use.

The second general manner in which livestock water can be contaminated during flooding is usually limited to coastal areas. Storm surges may bring brackish water or seawater into contact with shallow-well and surface water sources for livestock. Nontraumatized animals usually avoid brackish water or seawater. In most cases, healthy animals are not at great risk for dehydration within the first 48 hours of water deprivation (CB Navarre, Louisiana State University, Baton Rouge, LA, personal communication, 2017). Conversely, dehydrated animals may drink highly salinized water out of desperation and, in so doing, further exacerbate dehydration. Surviving animals in such condition should be prevented from accessing salt-contaminated water sources and gradually transitioned to a fresh water source. This is best achieved by supplying frequent (ie, every 1–3 hours) small (ie, 0.5–2 gallon) water deliveries in such a manner that all affected animals confined together can drink at the same time.

Salt content of livestock water following a storm surge should be tested to determine safety. Salinity testing is usually available through University Extension, the Natural Resource Conservation Service, US Armed Forces, and other disaster-relief agencies. Results of salinity testing should be interpreted in light of the following guidelines[4]:

- Greater than 10,000 ppm (or mg/L): unsafe for all classes of cattle (note that 10,000 ppm = 1%)
- 7000 to 10,000 ppm: unsafe for pregnant and lactating cows, young calves, and heat-stressed cattle; potentially safe for mature nonpregnant, nonlactating, nonstressed cattle
- 5000 to 7000 ppm: safe for most classes of cattle; potentially unsafe for pregnant or lactating females
- 1000 to 5000 ppm: generally safe for all classes of cattle; however, diarrhea may result
- Less than 1000 ppm: safe for all classes of cattle

Grain and forage resources that come into contact with floodwaters can be affected in all of the same ways that water sources can be affected. An additional challenge with livestock feedstuffs that become wet is subsequent growth of molds that can put human and animal health at risk. Preserved forages (eg, hay bales and silage) should be carefully examined for obvious generation of heat or the presence of molds. Examinations of this nature should only be performed by persons wearing gloves, coveralls, eye googles, and a respiration mask. Some molds may become airborne when forages are being examined and can be inhaled to the detriment of animal caregivers.

Forage sources that are hot to the touch should be considered at risk for spontaneous combustion. If possible, they should be moved away from structures and other valuable properties to a location where they can be thoroughly spread out to minimize fire risks. Dangerously molded hay or silage will contain obvious white, gray, brown, or black plaques, especially in the interior of the forage mass; it may also carry an uncharacteristically sweet odor. Affected forages may appear dusty when the mass is broken apart or otherwise disturbed. Forages that are obviously moldy will normally be avoided by horses or ruminant livestock; however, hungry animals will consume them. In the case of necessity, certain precautions can be taken to reduce risks associated with feeding moldy forages to livestock.

Moldy forages should never be fed to horses because of the relatively high risk of colic and heaves. Similarly, moldy forages should never be fed to pregnant or lactating cattle. Inhalation of mold spores by pregnant or lactating dams may cause mycotic pneumonia, which has been implicated in late-term abortion, associated retained placenta, and mastitis. Certain molds can also be passed via milk to human and animal consumers.

In contrast, moldy forages may be fed to nonpregnant and growing cattle without major negative outcomes. Care should be taken to discard discolored or extremely dusty portions of the forage mass. Less affected portions should be offered to cattle after thorough mixing with noncontaminated feedstuffs. In the opinion of the authors, the ratio of moldy forage to nonmoldy forage in rations for nonpregnant, nonlactating ruminants should not exceed 25:75.

Moldy grains carry the same risks to livestock as moldy forages; therefore, similar precautions for flood-affected grains should be observed. A major difference between the 2 is that grains that have come into contact with water may be more salvageable than forages when conditions allow. Grain storage structures partially submerged by flood waters can be evacuated from the top via vacuum until moist grain is encountered. Obviously moist grain should be discarded, especially if it carries an odor of fermentation. Recovered and salvageable grains should be dried mechanically or spread out in the sun to a depth of 3 to 6 inches. Drying should continue until a moisture content $\leq 14\%$ is reached. Molds are not necessarily eliminated during drying. Feeding salvaged grains to horses and pregnant or lactating cattle should be avoided. For nonpregnant, nonlactating cattle, flood-affected grains should be diluted 25:75 with clean grain in rations.

An additional consideration for flood-affected forages and grains is the potential presence of metallic foreign material. If inadvertently ingested by livestock, metallic objects can puncture the gastrointestinal tract and lead to peritonitis. To improve safety of any feedstuffs suspected of being contaminated by metallic debris, they should be processed or fed using machinery that is equipped with magnets in whatever location the feedstuffs are discharged from processing equipment, feed mixing equipment, or milling machinery.

It should be noted that pastures inundated by flood waters may contain debris or other residues harmful to livestock. Pastures and fences should be inspected following a flood event, with particular attention paid to the area where drainage occurs. Flood debris and decaying organic matter should be removed and fences repaired before readmitting livestock. Saturated soils are at risk for compaction by hoof traffic; moreover, forage plants stressed by inundation or saltwater exposure should be allowed 30 days of rest before grazing is resumed.

## EMERGENCY FEEDING DURING BLIZZARDS

Beef cattle producers typically have advance warning with regard to winter storms, which allows producers to make advance preparations. Preparations often include staging feedstuffs in readily accessible locations or creating temporary windbreaks. The duration and magnitude of a winter storm often vary greatly across the impacted region. The ability of beef cattle to survive and cope with blizzard conditions is a function of both environmental conditions (ie, wind chill, precipitation, and humidity), access to shelter, and animal acclimation (ie, hair coat, tissue insulation, and body condition). In general, maintenance energy requirements increase approximately 1% for each degree below the temperature at which cattle begin experiencing cold stress. In wet conditions or when cattle have a hair coat typical of summer, cattle can begin experiencing cold stress at 15°C (59°F). In contrast, cattle with a dry winter hair coat experience cold stress at approximately −8.0°C (18°F).[5] Cold stress increases maintenance energy requirements but does not impact protein, mineral, or vitamin requirements. Cattle will consume snow and ice to meet their needs for water during blizzard conditions; thus, water is not as great of a concern. Conversely, cattle that are not accustomed to consuming snow may be hesitant to do so. Keep in mind that body heat must be expended in order to melt ingested snow and ice, which increases the degree of thermal stress placed on the animal. The most vulnerable animals are typically those maintained in open, extensive environments, such as native range, wheat pasture, or crop-residue fields. The classic response to cold stress in confinement situations is an increase in voluntary intake typically preceding the event; however, it has been documented that beef cows maintained in extensive environments spend less time grazing as temperatures decline below freezing and may not be able to graze snow-covered pastures.[6] Less grazing time effectively reduces forage intake and makes the challenge of meeting the nutrient requirements of the cattle even greater. The traditional production response to a cold weather event is to feed more of the current protein supplement being used or offer a greater amount of low-quality hay. Although the additional supplement and hay provided increase energy supply, it may not necessarily supply sufficient energy to meet the additional caloric demands associated with cold stress. Therefore, cattle experiencing cold stress should be fed relatively higher-quality hay than the basal forage or an additional small amount of grain in combination with the normal ration of protein supplement.

## EMERGENCY FEEDING FOLLOWING WILDFIRE

Maintaining cattle immediately following wildfire is challenging because of the lack of available feedstuffs, because both grazed and harvested forages are generally diminished. Dehydrated cattle will voluntarily consume ash-contaminated sources of water but should not be allowed to do so if preventable; ash may contain a variety of toxic contaminants.

Cattle are often moved to temporary confinement situations or allowed to graze nonburned available forage resources (typically lush, green forages that did not ignite). Cattle abruptly turned out on lush green forages, especially mature, lactating cows, may be at risk for hypomagnesemia or "grass tetany," a condition characterized by low blood magnesium and associated with grazing lush, green, fertilized, cool-season grasses or small cereal grain pastures (wheat, barley, triticale) during the winter months.[7] The magnesium concentration in forages of this type typically meets or exceeds the requirements of grazing livestock, but the potassium concentration is usually well above that required by grazing livestock; moreover, sodium is usually well below the needs of grazing livestock. The absorption of magnesium from the rumen is dramatically reduced in the presence of excess potassium and low sodium. The concentration of potassium in saliva and the rumen increase under conditions in which sodium is limited.[8] Therefore, it is recommended that cattle abruptly relocated to lush, fertilized forages be provided ample access to loose stock salt. Salt may be force fed if not readily consumed by top-dressing or hand-blending salt with concentrate feeds. The result is 2-fold: magnesium is absorbed with greater efficiency from the rumen, and potassium absorption from the rumen is diminished. Animal care providers should be cautioned against trying to provide greater amounts of magnesium directly in the form of a self-fed mineral supplement. Although this can be a viable means to address hypomagnesemia, inorganic sources of magnesium (eg, magnesium oxide) tend to be bitter. Consumption of supplemental inorganic magnesium may be inadequate unless it is blended with a palatable grain source, such as dried distiller's grain, soybean meal, or dried molasses.

Cattle will consume smoke-damaged hay, silage, and wet distiller's grain but do not appear to prefer them. Smoke-damaged feedstuffs should be offered in limited quantities or diluted with clean feedstuffs when possible. Grinding smoke-damaged hay may help disperse the smoke smell and appears to moderately improve palatability. Feeding fiber-based energy sources (eg, dried distiller's grains, corn gluten feed, or soybean hulls) or starch-based energy sources (eg, corn, sorghum, barley, or wheat) should be considered for cattle confined temporarily. The caloric density of fiber and starch-based concentrates are usually greater than that of hay; thus, the energy requirements of more animals can be met with less delivered feed when concentrates are used in combination with hay. Cattle can be successfully maintained on concentrate-based diets that contain only 10% to 20% roughages. The nutrition and management of confined cattle require special attention. Cattle producers should seek the advice of University Extension or nutrition professionals to ensure that animal nutrient requirements are met and the appropriate amount of roughage is provided.

Following wildfire, pasture resources require rest before livestock grazing can be reinitiated. Forage yields after wildfire can be diminished. This is generally not the case when wildfires occur in the spring during years with normal precipitation.[9] In contrast, wildfires that occur during drought conditions, during the dormant season, or upon sensitive soil types (eg, sandy soil) can be expected to diminish yields and effective carrying capacities for 1 or more years. The authors suggest a conservative approach to restocking after wildfire. The following summary is adapted from a Kansas State University publication[9]:

- The length of grazing bouts is generally simpler to manage that the number of animals allowed to graze a given pasture or range. Pay close attention to forage availability and end grazing at or before 50% of peak production has been removed.
- In locations with claypan soils and adequate rainfall, stocking rates during the year following wildfire should be 75% to 100% of normal (depending on forage yield). Stocking rates can be returned to normal the second year following wildfire.
- In locations with loamy, finely textured soils, stocking rates in the year following wildfire should be reduced to 65% to 70% of normal. In the second year following wildfire, stocking rates can be increased to 90% to 100% of prefire levels.
- In locations that are drought prone or with coarsely textured, sandy soils, stocking rates in the year following wildfire should be reduced to 25% to 50% of normal. Stocking rates may be increased to 50% to 75% of normal in the second year following wildfire and returned to normal during year 3.

## REFERENCES

1. McCollum FT III. Some points to consider about cattle water. 2010. Available at: http://amarillo.tamu.edu/files/2010/10/Some-points-to-consider-about-cattle-water. pdf. Accessed October 3, 2017.
2. National Academies of Sciences, Engineering, and Medicine. Nutrient requirements of beef cattle. 8th revised edition. Washington, DC: National Academies Press; 2016.

3. Mathis CP, Sawyer JE. Nutritional management of grazing beef cows. Vet Clin North Am Food Anim Pract 2007;23:1–19.
4. Wright CL. Management of water quality for cattle. Vet Clin North Am Food Anim Pract 2007;23:91–103.
5. Ames DR. Adjusting rations for climate. Vet Clin North Am Food Anim Pract 1988;4: 543–50.
6. Adams DC, Nelsen TC, Reynolds WL, et al. Winter grazing activity and forage intake of range cows in the northern great plains. J Anim Sci 1986;62:1240–6.
7. Stewart AJ, Vaughan JT. Hypomagnesemic tetany in cattle and sheep. In: Merck veterinary manual. 2016. Available at: http://www.merckvetmanual.com/metabolic-disorders/disorders-of-magnesium-metabolism/hypomagnesemic-tetany-in-cattle-and-sheep. Accessed November 27, 2017.
8. Underwood EJ, Suttle NF. Magnesium. In: The mineral nutrition of livestock. 3rd edition. Cambridge (England): CABI Publishing; 1999. p. 149–84.
9. Fick WH. Rangeland management following wildfire. Kansas State Agric. Exp. Sta. Publ. L514. Available at: https://www.bookstore.ksre.ksu.edu/pubs/l514.pdf. Accessed November 28, 2017.

# Tornado Preparation and Response in Feedlot Cattle

Samantha L. Boyajian, BS[a], Nels N. Lindberg, DVM[b],*, David P. Gnad, DVM, MS[c,1]

## KEYWORDS

• Emergency protocols • Disaster strike • Tornado • Natural disasters

## KEY POINTS

• Encouraging operations to develop emergency protocols is one of the best steps one can take as a veterinarian who may be called upon to help once disaster strikes.
• Poor plans yield slow progress, and in times of tornado damage, efficiency in recovery is critical for an operation.
• A veterinarian is a key player in animal stewardship as well as human health and safety during natural disasters.

## INTRODUCTION

Tornado Alley is a colloquial term given to the rough outlines in the central United States where tornado occurrences are disproportionately higher than in other regions. The alley overlies states like Texas, Nebraska, and Kansas, which are also the top 3 states with the highest cattle population in feedlots, respectively.[a] This combination leads to emergency situations that occur on an annual basis, usually during late spring to early fall. When disasters like tornadoes strike, a plan and protocol are absolutely necessary in order to handle these situations as efficiently as possible. Beef producers need a leadership team that is equipped and prepared to delegate and lead solutions to all problems that arise in the wake of a tornado. And that is where a veterinarian comes in.

## IMMEDIATE ASSESSMENT

In the first few hours after a tornado has hit, it is critical that the leadership team meets to discuss the initial triage plan. The leadership team would ideally be present on the

The authors have nothing to disclose.
[a] College of Veterinary Medicine, Kansas State University, 1700 Denison Avenue, Manhattan, KS 66502, USA; [b] Production Animal Consultation, 622 McKinley Street, Great Bend, KS 67530, USA; [c] Nebraska Veterinary Services, 450 East Deere Street, West Point, NE 68788, USA
[1] Present address: Great Bend, KS.
* Corresponding author.
E-mail address: nnlindberg@yahoo.com

[a] http://www.beefusa.org/beefindustrystatistics.aspx.

property in order to best assess the extent of damage both to animals and the facility itself. The team may consist of the feedlot owner, operation manager, veterinarian, nutritionist, attorney, insurance agent, and nutrient management professional. This list is not exhaustive and will need to be tailored to each different situation and feedlot. The key is to make sure the leadership team can address and develop plans for all areas affected by the tornado. Without a predesignated leadership team, immediate action will be delayed, and recovery efficiency may be affected.

In many cases, large numbers of volunteers will arrive to extend support and help. It is the author's experience that this work force can be of great value if the leadership team can effectively coordinate and lead the volunteer workforce. Alternatively, a large number of volunteers can create congestion and have a negative affect if they are not directed with a coordinated plan. Volunteers may be given tasks that are not necessarily animal-centered; therefore, cattle experience is not needed. Picking up debris throughout fields, for instance, can be designated to volunteers while feed crews and cowboy crews focus on other pressing matters related to their own expertise. It is important that the leadership team continually assess and address the risk for human safety.

Initially, depending on damage, the leadership team should determine if all animals are confined, and if not, what is the best way to confine to secure their safety as well as the general public? While the animal is being confined, an assessment can be made on animal health. The leadership team will want to develop a plan for euthanasia, treatment, relocation, and humane slaughter. Access to water and feed for animals will potentially be compromised; therefore, bringing in temporary water tanks and feed bunks may be needed during the first few days. The authors recommend that the leadership team comes together at least once a day to best streamline the response and keep recovery as efficient as possible. Conducting a team meeting once a day, ideally in the morning to update and prepare for the days' work ahead, is recommended to keep all employees and volunteers on the same page with the leadership team. There are many moving parts to recovery and repair of an operation that has been disabled by a tornado; these parts can quickly become disjointed without a smooth connection that keeps all parties involved and informed every day. Communication is an invaluable key in hectic situations like these and should not be a skipped step.

## CREATE A PROTOCOL

Developing a protocol that is tailored to the operation is essential, although it might seem tedious. Having a game plan allows the team to be as prepared as possible if a catastrophic event occurs. A disaster plan may not be perfect depending on the event, but it will position the operation to address the situation proactively.

A good place to start when developing a protocol from the ground up is to figuratively go around the premises and determine what the actions would be if different pieces of the facility were compromised. For example, prearrange how to respond to no electricity that prevents the feed mill from operating, or decide where to treat cattle if the hospital pen or barn is destroyed. By doing this, it will help tailor a protocol to fit with each specific operation and its own unique layout and facilities.

Along with deciding what to do with physical damage to facilities, the protocol should outline decisions that have been predetermined for potential situations, like media control leadership. Determining a point person to control any and all information going to outside sources will help ensure there is only 1 outlet while allowing others to keep their attention fully on their own designated duties. Along with media control, the protocol should also include individuals or teams that are in charge of the immediate needs such as water and feed acquisition and its containment. One of the first steps that will be addressed once recovery begins will be making these basic needs available to the animals. Pens can potentially be destroyed during a tornado; therefore, fencing or temporary pens may need to be created for animal containment and the procurement of the labor force associated with it would be best if outlined in advance.

One of the most pressing matters will be to triage injured animals, creating the plan of how decisions will be made and the chain of command for making the decisions such as euthanasia, treatment, relocation, and humane slaughter. It is difficult to predict injuries, but determining how to conduct euthanasia as well as the team needed to carry out euthanasia on a large scale is important. Clearly, the veterinarian will be critical in determining how to best handle injured animals. That being said, there may be other factors that influence decision making such as availability of transportation, access to humane slaughter facilities, and proximity to relocation facilities, underscoring the importance of the leadership team's communication and plan. Once the criteria for euthanasia have been determined, the goal should be to perform euthanasia as quickly and efficiently as possible, thereby minimizing animal suffering. If firearms are required for euthanasia, it is imperative to address the issue of humane safety. As mentioned, many times animal confinement may be compromised, and volunteers are present to provide labor support. This will likely slow the rate at which euthanasia can be performed, so multiple teams may be needed in large-scale catastrophes. After all cattle that require euthanasia have been humanely handled, a protocol should outline how to address the potentially large number of injured cattle. Injuries from flying shrapnel are not common in the feedlot setting, so specific treatment plans will be needed outside of the typical feedlot disease treatment protocols. Many injuries can be subclinical, and cattle may be sorted into healthy groups on initial assessment. Continuous reevaluation of cattle that were exposed to the tornado is important so originally undetected injuries or disease can be identified early and treated effectively.

An operation that has a protocol distributed to all of its employees and consulting professionals (eg, veterinarian and nutritionist) yields an efficient response to disasters. Being prepared in this manner pays off during a time when it is best to start working rather than waste precious hours trying to develop a plan on the spot. It cannot be stressed enough that a relevant protocol that is updated and well-known can truly save an operation valuable resources, time, and lives.

A protocol of this nature is strongly recommended for any operation, no matter its size, but creating a protocol is not the only step a feedlot can take to better prepare itself for tornado damage. One of the best ways to have an efficient reaction after a tornado has hit is to be prepared for the actual tornado itself. It's imperative to stay up to date on weather predictions during tornado season. This seems overly simplified, but each tornado season can provide another chance to revisit protocols or allow managers to conduct a recount of resources or supplies that may be needed should a tornado cause damage to the operation. By knowing the chance of high winds and tornado formation, operations can prepare ahead of time to the best of their ability in anticipation of bad weather.

## EXECUTION

An operation that has a well thought out protocol and has kept up to date with personnel changes will have an execution phase that will be as smooth as can be expected.

### Safety

Downed power lines are a common problem associated with tornado damage. Ensuring someone on the leadership team reaches out to the city or county energy provider in charge of shutting down power to those lines is essential before damage management can really be underway. Human safety should always be kept at the forefront of the response and that includes animals that may no longer be confined to pens. Some cattle will likely be disoriented during the initial hours after the disaster but can become fractious and difficult to handle as time continues. This poses a threat to all who are working to repair the operation, especially volunteers who may not be able to safely assess reactions from the animals. This is why the animal team in charge of welfare should be confining animals during the euthanasia and treatment phases.

## Animal Care

The practice of euthanasia can take much longer than it needs to and can be shortened if the beginning of the process is aligned to a protocol. The procedure itself may theoretically appear to be simple, but underestimating the time, resources, or human labor involved with euthanasia can make this task more difficult than it needs to be. First response should be to sort animals into pens for treatment if euthanasia on the spot is not warranted. It is good to note that standard euthanasia practices may not be practical in these scenarios, because pens and chutes may be disabled. Therefore, euthanasia may need to take place in an open field or in the home pen. Animals that are sorted into treatment pens or confines can most likely be dealt with after those requiring euthanasia are attended to. Many injuries will center around traumatic type injuries such as lacerations, punctures, and even fractures; however, it is possible for animals to have internal injuries that may appear clinically normal. For the days and weeks to follow, it is recommended to ask crews to remain intentionally focused on all animals, as often times animals with injuries may be nonclinical immediately following a tornado but with time and fulmination of an injury become clinical days to weeks after the weather event.

## Water

This is a step that is easily overlooked during the chaos of repairs, unconfined animals, and power outages, but it is a crucial step that needs addressed. Both for animals and people working long days, make sure fresh water is available. This may require having water brought in from other facilities or operations, because the water source could be compromised, especially if it was run by electricity, such as automatic water tanks. Have a team specifically tasked with providing a water source, maintaining that water accessibility, and finding a new area to hold water if necessary.

## Feed

The nutritionist can determine if the feed source has been compromised. If the mill has been damaged, then this will need to be addressed much like the water situation by assessing options for feed. Options can be bringing in a portable roller mill to roll corn or procuring rolled corn or flaked corn from another operation or facility until the mill is fully repaired and operational. Along with ensuring feed is still available on the property it will be necessary to check bunk integrity or creating temporary bunks for new pens that animals are held in if the original pens were destroyed.

## Carcass Removal

Certain aspects will be nearly impossible to predict; some instances have required increased machinery just to move carcasses, and this need may be exacerbated by heat stress along with emergency dig sites. The weather is the focus for the start of the tornado, but realizing that the weather strongly affects the aftermath can help an operation be even more prepared. Given that tornado season overlaps with increased climate temperatures, severe heat stress can become an enormous piece of the treatment puzzle. Knowing ahead of time the operation's available emergency dig site, if needed, can save precious time rather than determining that information during the actual event.

### Missing Cattle

It will be imperative to maintain records as the veterinarian begins euthanizing and treating animals, not only for insurance and withdrawal purposes but to also ensure that all animals are accounted for. It will be fairly easy once fencing is destroyed for animals to become dislocated from their pens or even the feedlot property itself. As the animal team moves through to address injured animals and reorganize the pens, documenting and taking headcounts on affected pens or all pens are necessary to ensure appropriate head counts of pens are reconciled in the feedlot accounting software, between cattle in the home pen, cattle in the hospital or recovery pens, cattle euthanized, cattle relocated, and cattle missing.

### Horses

Although livestock and people tend to be the main focus in these events, it is also recommended to ensure that horse welfare is observed and assessed and treatments rendered as needed. Horses are an important piece to the success of day-to-day operations as well as in response to a disaster, so their continued health and wellbeing are critical. Much like cattle, the common health issues associated with tornado events are injuries such as laceration and fractures; therefore, they should be triaged and treated accordingly. Repair of or providing alternative housing for horses may be needed.

### Media Control

Part of the leadership team that should be predetermined in the protocol is the media point person. Ideally this position has been predesignated, but if not then it should be determined quickly. Media are typically attracted to disasters, and if large numbers of animals are affected, the likelihood of media attention increases. It is important that a concise, accurate message be communicated to the media to prevent misinformation or sensationalizing. A short list of bullet points can be prepared quickly to focus on the important elements of the recovery process. The following are examples of bullet points that have been used by the authors:

- We are working very hard to care for all affected animals.
- The safety of people working to care for the animals is of utmost importance to us.
- Animals that are injured are being treated and cared for.

### Communication

One of the most important aspects during the execution of tornado recovery on an operation is to stick with the written protocol and keep communication at the top of the priority list. These 2 keys help the most during a time when chaos can quickly take hold of an ill-prepared operation. All personnel should meet once a day to exchange updates or make any changes to the existing protocol if the current event requires it. As a veterinarian and a key consultant for an operation of any size, developing a protocol with the actual execution in mind keeps it relevant and applicable. Unintended consequences and unforeseen circumstances will arise, thus the need for once-a-day meetings to address these issues. Protocols are a wonderful tool to aid in preparation, keep people on the same page with the plan, reduce confusion, and provide clarity, although protocols must be flexible to fit the needs of the operation at the specific point in time given the weather, personnel involved, and all the extreme variables in a feeding operation.

## SUMMARY

Encouraging operations to develop these emergency protocols is one of the best steps one can take as a veterinarian who may be called upon to help once disaster strikes. Poor plans yield slow progress, and in times of tornado damage, efficiency in recovery is critical for an operation. A veterinarian is a key player in animal stewardship as well as human health and safety during natural disasters. The veterinarian should be an integral part in the planning so that he or she can be prepared to be a valuable part in the recovery.

# Blizzards and Range Cattle

## Management Before, During, and After the Storm

Russ Daly, DVM, MS[a],*, Cynthia Marshall Faux, DVM, PhD[b]

### KEYWORDS

- Blizzard • Cattle • Calving • Weaning • Frostbite

### KEY POINTS

- Severe winter storms and blizzards are infrequent but potentially devastating aspects of livestock production in temperate parts of the world.
- Mitigation practices that have protected cattle and improved recovery of lost cattle include animal identification, identification of shelter, and understanding behavior in a storm.
- Timing of the storm within the production cycle presents different challenges (eg, calving).
- The ability of the producer and emergency management to facilitate post-storm care and rescue can mitigate losses, but large numbers of animal casualties can be expected from major storms.
- Animal behavior may be altered after the storm and rescue and production practices may require accommodation for these concerns.

## INTRODUCTION

For as long as cattle have been domesticated in temperate areas of the world, severe winter storms and blizzards have wreaked havoc on cattle herds. Reports from the 1800s and early 1900s describe losses of thousands of cattle during such storms and likely forced changes in cattle producers' "open range" methods of cattle rearing.[1,2] Recently, the scope and devastation of blizzards on cattle herds have been no less significant, despite modern cattle management methods available to producers.[3–5] An April, 2017, blizzard killed "thousands" of cattle in Colorado, Kansas, and Oklahoma,[3,5] a blizzard in December 2015 was responsible for 12,000 dead cattle

The authors have nothing to disclose.
[a] Department of Veterinary and Biomedical Science, South Dakota State University, Box 2175, Brookings, SD 57007, USA; [b] Department of Integrated Physiology and Neurosciences, Washington State University College of Veterinary Medicine, Veterinary and Biomedical Research Building, Room 205, Washington State University, Pullman, WA 99164-7620, USA
* Corresponding author.
*E-mail address:* russell.daly@sdstate.edu

in the Texas Panhandle,[6] and an early season South Dakota blizzard was blamed for killing 25,000 animals.[4]

Additionally, winter storms result in a myriad of health problems for the survivors in the herd, as well as management problems for cattle producers. Learning from the experiences of these recent events can be instructive as cattle producers, veterinarians, and emergency personnel prepare for, respond, and recover from these extreme weather events.

## PREPARATIONS BEFORE A BLIZZARD

A blizzard warning may provide a very narrow window of opportunity, several days at most, for preparation before a storm. Certain routine management practices, implemented by cattle producers well in advance of a blizzard, can prove very valuable in mitigating the impact of severe winter weather on their cattle.

### Animal Identification

Perhaps the one management procedure that has, in retrospect, benefited cattle producers the most after severe blizzards has been that of effective animal identification. In the aftermath of recent severe blizzards, cattle have been found long distances from their origin and, owing to their natural herd instincts, will often become comingled with other groups of cattle they may encounter during a storm. Those herds with existing suitable animal identification were more likely to recover the maximum number of strayed cattle. Sufficient animal identification is not something that can be easily implemented in the day or two before a winter storm. Cattle fitted with ear tags that are unique to the herd of origin and easily visualized, especially from a distance, can be more easily matched to a specific herd. Brands are also unique herd identifiers, but have limitations of legibility, especially on cattle in winter hair. Brands may also be difficult for community laypeople assisting with recovery efforts to identify and interpret.

### Sheltering

Given enough lead time, producers can attempt to move animals closer to shelter and feed sources when possible. Windbreaks and the outside walls of buildings may provide some shelter from wind and driving snow. In severe and prolonged winter storms, however, past experience has shown that this measure will not always preclude animals from straying away from these sheltered areas during the storm.

With smaller groups of cattle and larger available sheds, producers may opt to shelter their cattle inside or allow them access to such shelter. The available space offered by buildings should be evaluated critically with regard to herd numbers. In particular, crowding of cow/calf pairs inside a building for prolonged periods can result in serious injuries to young calves if they are stepped on or crushed by the cows.[7]

Sheds or buildings should have adequate ventilation for the number of housed animals. Overheating and respiratory issues in animals of all ages, owing to insufficient ventilation, may be a sequela to prolonged periods of shelter in buildings. Open-front sheds with slot openings underneath the eaves on the back wall will provide for some airflow, improve ventilation, and may prevent excessive snow from piling up in front of the shed.[7]

Heavy snowfall in some recent blizzards has resulted in the collapse of such buildings.[8] Heavy snowfall, especially when the snow is wet, may completely consume buildings housing cattle, resulting in suffocation. This possibility should be considered when making the difficult decision of whether to house cattle during a blizzard.

**RESPONSE**
*During a Blizzard*

Moving cattle during blizzards, even if human safety is ensured, can prove problematic. Cattle tend to resist traveling into winds. In addition, their normal survival instincts may make them hesitant to leave areas where they have even rudimentary shelter. Travel over areas of poor footing or into unfamiliar areas may also make moving groups of cattle more challenging.[7]

Cattle that are not satisfied with their shelter during a blizzard can be expected to drift with the prevailing wind direction. Cattle may find temporary shelter in draws, canyons, ravines, and similar microhabitats, especially if they are familiar with those locations. These areas may provide sufficient protection if the snow event is not heavy or prolonged.

Cattle have wandered great distances from their home base; stocker cattle were found 70 miles from their home pasture, having walked that far during and after a recent Texas blizzard.[3] During the course of a prolonged storm, wind directions usually shift and the cattle may continue to move accordingly, in a nonlinear pattern. As described, cattle may find shelter in draws or ravines. However, during heavy prolonged blizzards, cattle in such locations have been snowed in or drifted under, leading to their suffocation.[9] Heavy snowfall and drifting may bury fences, allowing animals to walk over or become entangled in them. Power outages may allow animals to breach electric fences they would not otherwise challenge.

*The Immediate Aftermath*

Although every blizzard is unique in its scope and severity, veterinarians, cattle producers, and emergency responders can heed the lessons learned from previous storms to inform preparedness and response plans.

Impassable roads are a critical factor affecting the response to a blizzard once the snow and winds subside. Blocked roads make it difficult or impossible to search for stray cattle, to transport strayed animals home, or to supply feed to animals stranded in remote locations. Although cattle producers (or their neighbors) may have on-farm snow blowers and loaders that can be used to dig out driveways and private roads, access to some remote areas may not be possible for several days or more. Producers' priorities should initially lie in restoring access to main roads so people can get to the nearest town for supplies and, if needed, emergency services.

Power outages owing to the blizzard may further complicate efforts to care for cattle and hinder communications.

Those finding cattle in the aftermath of a blizzard usually find those animals in 1 of 4 circumstances:

1. Cattle that are able to ambulate and travel normally.
2. Cattle that are alive and trapped by fences, snowdrifts, in creek bottoms, and so on, but otherwise ambulatory.
3. Cattle that are alive but unable to travel because of injury or exhaustion.
4. Dead cattle.

*Rescuing trapped animals*

Before attempting any individual animal extrication or rescue effort, responders encountering trapped cattle should make an accurate assessment of the health condition of the animal. Severe exhaustion and hypothermia (rectal temperatures below 82°F) may warrant immediate euthanasia (see Jan K. Shearer and colleagues' article, "Humane Euthanasia and Carcass Disposal," in this issue) unless it is possible to provide a source of external warmth to the animal.[10] Assessment for injuries, especially to those cattle that are, or were, entangled in fences or other obstacles may indicate immediate euthanasia.

Before any extrication, rescuer safety is paramount. Many producers affected by the 2013 South Dakota blizzard observed aggressive behavior in surviving cattle, particularly older cattle. Aggressive behavior, anecdotally at least, has been ascribed to conditions of cerebral hypoxia. Hypothetically, cows that survived the blizzard but were affected by pulmonary edema or other circumstances impairing oxygenation might show aggressive behavior as a consequence. In addition, aggressive behavior has been noted in early cases of grass or transport tetany (discussed elsewhere in this article). Rescuers should, therefore, approach cattle with caution, and should take care to avoid getting kicked, butted, or run over while cutting fence or scooping snow close to these animals, as well as immediately upon the animal's freedom from the obstacle. The cow in a cow–calf pair should always be approached with caution.

When extracting a trapped animal, care should first be taken to remove any impediments for the animal to rise and walk. Fence wires may need to be cut to free the animal, and snow should be scooped away from the animal as well for a distance in front of the animal. If animals are unable to rise immediately, they should be allowed to rest without disturbance for a period of time, up to several hours, to allow them to regain their energy, and then reevaluated. If the animal is still nonambulatory, options including euthanasia or transport to a more sheltered area for further care should be considered.

When animals are caught in snowbanks, in deep draws, or stuck in mud surrounding stock dams or creek beds, more active means of extrication may be necessary. Regardless of the situation, rescuers should adhere to principles of humane movement of nonambulatory animals.[11] Direct attachment of chains, cables, or tow ropes to the neck, limbs, or tail should be avoided. Whenever at all feasible, cattle should be placed on mats or sleds and moved in that manner. Hip lifts and slings can be used to position animals on these conveyances, but not used to directly move animals.[11]

### Managing displaced cattle

Roads rendered impassable by snow or mud make it challenging to retrieve cattle and return them to their home base. Therefore, groups of cattle may need to "shelter in place" for several days while conditions allow trucks, trailers, and corral panels to arrive at the location. When encountering groups of displaced cattle, rescuers may need to improvise methods of confinement. For example, in a recent blizzard, a group of cattle was herded into, and confined on, a baseball field.[12]

As mentioned, prior animal identification is of extreme value in returning animals to their herd of origin. Ear tags unique to individual herds (eg, a particular tag color, or with producer contact information) are simple to recognize and identify by a wide variety of first responders. Brands can be effective in matching cattle to herds, but are more difficult for non–cattle producers to describe or identify.

In recent blizzards involving animals that strayed long distances, social media platforms have proved valuable in communicating the number, type, and location of displaced cattle.[12] Facebook pages have been created where responders posted pictures and descriptions of found cattle. Producers could monitor these sites and easily communicate with those who found the cattle. Current technology allows this communication to take place via smartphones directly at the location of the animals.

Local officials and cattle producers may need to coordinate temporary feed and water sources for these displaced cattle, especially when they have found shelter in unconventional locales. Scene evaluation is essential because, even in the face of deep snowfall, cattle may find adequate forage. For example, after the 2013 South Dakota early fall storm, cattle had immediate access to reasonable quality forage, because large expanses of rangeland on ridges and hilltops had been blown clear of snow.

In cases where groups of cattle are found isolated on remote pastures, local officials may find it necessary to consider "hay drops" to provide these animals with temporary life-saving nutrition.[13] Cattle can use snow for a water source for short periods of times in emergencies[14]; however, a lack of feed over several days—especially in cold conditions—can rapidly deplete existing energy stores, particularly in cows already in poor condition or in younger animals.

Immediately after the Colorado blizzards in 1997 and 2007, emergency management officials coordinated hay drops via aircraft—and eventually land vehicles—for cattle cut off from feed sources. In those cases, state officials relied on the cooperative efforts of a long list of entities to ensure that feed was delivered to animals in need. State and county emergency management operation centers, state departments of agriculture and transportation, the Civil Air Patrol, the National Guard, and independent contractors coordinated efforts to deliver hay to stranded cattle. In addition, the state veterinarian's office, university extension, and local and state livestock producer groups coordinated to identify and provide contact information for ranchers in the affected area who may need assistance.[15] Livestock producer groups should make themselves aware of, and become part of, formal state and county disaster response plans. For more information on feeding cattle during blizzards, please see J.W. Waggoner and K.C. Olson's article, "Feeding and Watering Beef Cattle During Disasters," in this issue.

*Cattle health issues*

Exposure to severe cold can result in hypothermia, even in adult cattle. Hypothermia can be exacerbated by wet haircoats and wind speeds. Mild clinical hypothermia can occur when body temperatures reach 86°F to 89°F, moderate hypothermia at 71°F to 85°F, with severe cases occurring when body temperatures drop to 68°F or below.[10] As rectal temperatures drop below 82°F, a cow cannot return to normal body temperature without some form of assistance, either through warming or administration of warm fluids.[10]

Whether the cattle succumb or survive a severe winter storm may depend on the obstacles they confront during their journey. In the 2013 South Dakota blizzard, cattle encountered many physical obstacles, unavoidable in the blinding snow and wind. Cattle were found in fence lines, especially in southeast and southwest corners of pastures, unable to cross them.[9]

Exhaustion is a common cause of death of cattle caught in blizzards, owing to their struggling to free themselves from snow drifts or muddy areas of rivers, dams, or creeks, or simply from the exertion put forth in miles of walking through wind and snow. Extreme physical exertion coupled with increased energy demands from wind chills results in animals becoming spent of energy and no longer able to walk. As such, many dead animals are not only found in fence lines, but others are found at or near the tops of ridges and hills, collapsed in place.[9]

Pulmonary changes have also been implicated as contributing to death in cattle in blizzards. Terminal pulmonary edema from left-sided heart failure has been proposed as a sequelae to extreme exhaustion and stress.[9]

In the 2013 South Dakota blizzard, several cases of a tetany-like condition, similar to grass tetany, were reported in animals immediately after the blizzard.[9] Animals were found in a hyperexcitable phase, progressing to recumbency and muscle tremors. Transport tetany and grass tetany produce similar clinical signs and this postblizzard syndrome may be related. Long-term (>24 hours) deprivation of feed and water and stress from transportation are considered major inciting factors for transport tetany. The specific causes of this syndrome are unclear; some observers postulate that acute hypocalcemia, hypomagnesemia, and physical stress are involved. Subsequent unrestricted access to feed and water precipitates clinical signs. Treatment is often unrewarding, but consists of intravenous administration of calcium–magnesium–glucose products.[16] Although cattle are not transported, per se, during blizzards, stress along with feed and water deprivation are often factors.

A similar syndrome that may have caused clinical signs in those blizzard affected cattle is grass tetany. This condition typically occurs on pasture when consumed forages are low in magnesium, and can also be exacerbated when weather conditions result in feeding disruptions. Rapid springtime pasture growth, with relatively cold soils, results in a lower magnesium content of forages and is typically associated with grass tetany. Cases of grass tetany have also been associated with rapid pasture growth in the fall when warm, moist conditions are present. Although not documented, low forage magnesium levels could have contributed to these signs of tetany after that early fall storm. Treatment of these cases also consists of calcium–magnesium–glucose infusions intravenously, and is often unrewarding. Prevention in spring and fall pasture situations involves use of high-magnesium mineral.[17]

Cases of bloating in nursing calves were observed in the days immediately after the 2013 South Dakota storm. The etiology of bloat in relation to the storm aftermath was unclear, but likely resulted from disruptions in feeding patterns, or—more likely—rapid resumption of feeding and resulting milk overload, or acidosis, when the storm was over. Rumen acidosis and the resulting ruminal dysfunction may have been a contributing factor for bloating. Most of these cases responded well to relief with a stomach tube and treatment with mineral oil, antacids, and similar medications.[9]

These metabolic and digestive disruptions in animals surviving blizzards should encourage discretion in allowing immediate access to high-quality feed and water after prolonged deprivation. Producers may, when possible, better serve their animals for the long term by considering restricting full access to high-quality alfalfa or concentrates immediately after the storm. Limit feeding and gradually increasing fed amounts and feed quality over several days may ward off some of the clinical signs noted herein. These feed management strategies are more applicable in situations when stranded animals have been returned home to their normal feedstocks, and less applicable when the emergency nutritional needs of animals stranded away from normal feedstocks in bitter environmental conditions must be considered. For more information on feeding cattle during blizzards, please see J.W. Waggoner and K.C. Olson's article, "Feeding and Watering Beef Cattle During Disasters," in this issue.

### Carcass management and disposal

After accounting for and caring for surviving animals, cattle producers and regulatory officials face the grim task of disposing of dead animals. Removal and disposal of all livestock carcasses may take a substantial amount of time in a blizzard's aftermath. People working to perform this task face many challenges, including the following.

- Winter temperatures and subsequent snowfall will make it hard to locate animals until after significant snow melt—days or weeks later.
- Animals that succumb to blizzard conditions may die in inaccessible locations, such as steep draws and ravines.

- Rendering services may not be available in all locations, or if they are, will be quickly overwhelmed.
- The sheer number of dead animals (perhaps in the tens of thousands) presents serious challenges to timely disposal.

Before dead cattle are moved, producers should take time to document each animal, including their location and ear tag numbers, along with photographs. The US Department of Agriculture, and potentially state agencies as well, may have livestock indemnity programs in place to assist cattle producers suffering losses. In a similar manner, those holding insurance policies covering cattle death owing to weather events should take care to document the death losses as well. It is recommended that producers contact these entities to determine what specific documentation is required before disposing of cattle and other livestock. Some entities will require third parties such as veterinarians, local extension personnel, and local county conservation district staff to verify and sign off on such records before they are considered valid. Producers should be encouraged to inquire about these requirements as well.

State and local animal disaster response plans should contain verbiage regarding carcass disposal, including contingencies. State and local officials should work to communicate, and producers and responders should seek to understand, pertinent regulations and response plans surrounding proper disposal of dead livestock. For example, in South Dakota, approved means of disposal include burning, burying, or rendering—normally within 48 hours of death. If a state considers individual producer plans for disposal of livestock mortalities by composting, the sheer numbers and sizes of animals lost in a widespread blizzard may preclude that as a practical means of disposal.

Responsibility for disposal of cattle finding their way onto public right of ways is also governed by local and state regulations. Although dead cattle found on private land and on private roadways are often the responsibility of the landowner, cattle found in county or state highway roadways are usually considered the responsibility of those entities.

Approved methods of livestock disposal are designed to mitigate any potential human health problems that may arise from dead carcasses. These methods mitigate the likelihood of carcasses attractiveness to wildlife scavengers such as coyotes or skunks. In addition, any animal euthanized via chemical means, such as barbiturates, requires carcass disposal by means that prevent scavenging. Harm to scavengers, such as eagles, carry severe legal penalties. Although the vast majority of animals succumbing to blizzards were healthy before death, healthy animals can occasionally harbor contagious or zoonotic agents. However, the expected concentration of these organisms (eg, *Salmonella, Campylobacter, Escherichia coli* O157:H7, and *Cryptosporidium*) in normal range cattle is very low. Cattle pathogens such as infectious bovine rhinotracheitis, bovine respiratory syncytial virus, and bovine viral diarrhea virus, which are not zoonotic, have a very short survival time outside a living animal. Although members of the public may become concerned about carcasses lying in waterways, even in the infrequent case in which animal carcasses harbor these agents, the flow of water in these waterways will tremendously dilute these pathogens, likely making the risk to animals or people downstream negligible.

Animal carcasses can contribute to poor water quality through the products of their decomposition (increased dissolved solids, increased biological oxygen demand, etc), so burial in close proximity to drinking water wells should be avoided. In the case of waterways, dilution through normal water flows typically means there is little to no effect on water quality downstream. Please refer to Jan K. Shearer and colleagues' article, "Humane Euthanasia and Carcass Disposal," in this issue, for additional information and discussion.

### Human safety issues

With catastrophic weather events, livestock producers are rightfully extremely concerned about the well-being of their animals. However, these concerns should not overshadow the need to consider the safety and well-being of people during the storm and its aftermath.

Beyond basic winter storm safety, cattle producers and emergency responders should take special care in the following situations unique to animal emergencies during and after blizzards.

- Avoiding injury (kicks, head butts, crushing) from animals while providing direct aid to them (digging out from snow, cutting loose from fences).
- Avoiding injury from vehicles and equipment used to move cattle (tractors, trailers, panels, etc).
- Recognizing that cattle may display unusual aggressive behavior after a storm.

In addition, responders and neighbors should be mindful of the extreme stress and mental health issues that may arise in people affected by these catastrophic events. Beside the obvious economic disaster producers face, one should not underestimate the bond between these caretakers and their animals. In past blizzards, years of valuable genetic progress, let alone some special "favorite" animals, have been wiped out in a matter of hours. All those involved should be aware of help lines and mental health resources available in the aftermath of these tragedies. Please refer to Erin Wasson and Audry Wieman's article, ""I Can't Stop Thinking About It": Mental Health During Environmental Crisis and Mass Incident Disasters," in this issue, for additional discussion.

The important role of local and state government and emergency personnel in response to widespread blizzard events cannot be overstated. In addition to the obvious responsibilities of clearing roads, restoring power, and search-and-rescue efforts for people stranded in the storms, these entities can provide valuable coordination and communication regarding the following.

- Communication with livestock producers in need of assistance in providing emergency feed for or locating lost cattle.
- Coordinating emergency feed deliveries to groups of cattle cut off from feed sources.
- Coordinating rendering services from outside the area.
- Designating and approving burial sites.

Please refer to Dee Ellis and colleagues' article, "Communication During Natural Disasters and Working with Authorities," in this issue, for more information on communication and working with authorities.

## RECOVERY
### Medium- to Long-Term Effects on Animals After Blizzards

An increase in bovine respiratory disease complex has been reported 7 to 14 days after a blizzard in susceptible calves.[9] Affected calves responded to veterinary treatment; however, group treatment of animals on range was difficult. An increase in pinkeye was observed in calves after a recent blizzard. The typical causative agents, *Moraxella bovis* and *Moraxella bovoculi*, generally require an inciting irritation, such as dust, to cause disease. In the case of the blizzard, it was postulated that driving snow and wind sufficiently irritated the animals' eyes to allow the establishment of disease. Affected animals responded to routine treatment protocols.[9]

Frostbite is a danger for exposed tissues, especially extremities. Ears, teats, the prepuce and scrotum, and feet are particularly at risk. The long-term consequences of frostbite include sloughing of tissue and subsequent scarring. Preputial scarring and stenosis can be severe enough to prevent penile extension and require surgical intervention to rectify. Freezing of the distal scrotum may result in scarring severe enough to raise the testicles within the scrotum close enough to the body to affect thermoregulation and, thus, fertility. Breeding soundness examinations of bulls should be undertaken.[18]

Winter storms may hit cattle operations at various stages of their management cycle—anytime from preweaning through calving, in spring calving herds, resulting in unique challenges and circumstances for these stages of management.

### Blizzards Occurring Before Weaning (Early Fall)

A blizzard occurring in early October 2013 in South Dakota illustrated some unique challenges of early season winter storms in the Midwest.[9] In that storm, many calves were still nursing and on pasture. These cattle were more likely to be on remote summer pastures. In storms occurring later in the winter, they would typically be housed closer to home and closer to shelter from winter winds and precipitation.

Early season storms are also more likely to begin with rain first, which then turns to snow. As a result, animals' hair coats are more likely to become saturated before temperatures decrease and wind speeds increase. This situation greatly exacerbates the onset of hypothermia in exposed cattle, because the insulating activity of the haircoat is lost. Additionally, if fall weather has previously been mild, cattle will not have developed their thicker winter hair coat, exacerbating the situation. Cattle in such a predicament direct more of their body energy stores to thermoregulation, putting them quickly into a state of negative energy balance. Compounding this state, a great proportion of cows involved in the October South Dakota blizzard were still nursing their calves, and therefore were already in relatively poor body condition.

The preceding rains of early season snowstorms—and the eventual temperature warm-up afterward—contribute to muddy conditions, which can become more of a concern during storm recovery. Such conditions can be as much of an impediment to transport and travel in pastures and gravel/dirt roads as the snow and ice.

When about-to-be-weaned calves are involved in a prolonged stressful storm, unique management challenges arise. Producers and veterinarians should examine the timing of any preweaning or weaning time vaccinations. Calves stressed from the storm and its aftermath, may have a poor vaccine response and it may be prudent to delay vaccinations, or other stressful procedures, until calves have sufficient time to recover from the weather event. The timing of late fall storms may prompt changes in calf marketing decisions, highlighting the need for flexibility. For example, in the early season South Dakota blizzard, producers who had historically been inclined to sell the calves immediately off the cow, opted to keep calves at home and on feed after weaning. Such producers may need guidance regarding feeding and facilities for backgrounding calves, if this was not previously a feature of the ranch operation.

### Blizzards Occurring During Calving Season

Late season blizzards bring their own set of challenges to cattle operations, particularly if they occur during calving season. Although animals are more likely to be closer to care and shelter during calving, the vulnerability of newborn calves to harsh winter weather presents its own set of difficult circumstances.

Calves born in frigid blizzard conditions are especially vulnerable to hypothermia. Chilled calves should be warmed by use of warming boxes, blankets, or warm water baths to maintain or increase their body temperature to greater than 94°F. In addition, care should be taken to ensure the calf has adequate colostrum during the first few hours of life; colostrum provides critical nutrients for the maintenance of body temperature.[19]

Young calves are also susceptible to frostbite when exposed to bitter cold temperatures and winds during a blizzard. Calves' extremities such as their ears, tails, and hind feet are commonly affected. Appropriate shelter and bedding during extreme cold and wind is the only true means of prevention; once evidence of frostbite is observed in a calf, tissue damage has already occurred. Directly applying warm water or towels to the affected extremities may help to limit the damage.[20] Frostbite is also a concern for the teats of heifers and cows exposed to extreme cold and wind, and therefore predisposes calves to not having access to colostrum or milk, with all the downstream effects of poor nutrition being compounded on the immediate cold weather concerns.

## SUMMARY

Numerous factors contribute to the outcome and recovery for range cattle affected by blizzard. Consequences and impact on the producer depend on the timing of the storm relative to the herd's production cycle (early preweaning vs calving season), access to shelter (whether man-made or natural protection), duration and intensity of the storm, and post-storm emergency management effectiveness. Critical planning efforts by the producer include clear animal identification methods, identification of sheltering options, and consideration of animal indemnity and insurance requirements. Including range animals in local and state disaster planning efforts facilitates response and recovery efforts. Response efforts must include understanding of postincident animal behavior concerns, such as animal aggression and entrapment, as well as producer and responder mental health.

## ACKNOWLEDGMENTS

The authors wish to thank Barrett Slenning, North Carolina State University, and Suzanne Fricke, Washington State University, for their suggestions and critical review of the article.

## REFERENCES

1. Clark L. The 1887 blizzard that changed the American Frontier Forever. Smithsonian.com 2015. Available at: https://www.smithsonianmag.com/smart-news/1887-blizzard-changed-american-frontier-forever-1-180953852/. Accessed November 27, 2017.

2. Pfankuch B. Which snowstorm was the worst in history? Here is a look back at some bad ones. Rapid City Journal 2013. Available at: http://rapidcityjournal.com/news/local/which-snowstorm-was-the-worst-in-history-here-is-a/article_62f9ee47-6889-5955-bfc7-d3f59e52d34f.html. Accessed November 7, 2017.

3. Bechtel W. Blizzard kills an estimated 12,000 beef cattle, another 40,000 missing. AgWeb News 2016. Available at: https://www.agweb.com/article/blizzard-kills-an-estimated-12000-beef-cattle-another-40000-missing-naa-wyatt-bechtel/. Accessed November 7, 2017.

4. Radke A. Early South Dakota blizzard leaves thousands of cattle dead. Beef Daily 2013. Available at: http://www.beefmagazine.com/blog/early-south-dakota-blizzard-leaves-thousands-cattle-dead. Accessed November 7, 2017.
5. Scott K. Ranchers assessing death loss, stray cattle location after snow storm. High Plains/Midwest Ag Journal 2017. Available at: http://www.hpj.com/livestock/ranchers-assessing-death-loss-stray-cattle-location-after-snow-storm/article_7caa5784-301b-11e7-b75b-ef0195cabd82.html. Accessed November 7, 2017.
6. Ledbetter K. Latent effects of blizzard a concern for cow-calf producers. Texas A&M AgriLife Today 2016. Available at: https://today.agrilife.org/2016/01/05/latent-effects-of-blizzard-a-concern-for-cow-calf-producers/. Accessed November 7, 2017.
7. Severe Cold Weather Rangeland and Livestock. Extension fact sheet, undated. Available at: http://extension.colostate.edu/topic-areas/agriculture/severe-cold-weather-rangeland-and-livestock-considerations/. Accessed November 27, 2017.
8. Naylor C. 1966 Blizzard takes toll on N.D. Ranchers, Livestock. 2016. Available at: http://www.kfyrtv.com/home/headlines/1966-Blizzard-Takes-Toll-on-ND-Ranchers-Livestock-370841941.html. Accessed November 27, 2017.
9. Daly R, Olson K, Ollila D, et al. Animal health effects of the October 2013 blizzard: observations. In Proceedings of The Range Beef Cow Symposium XXIII. Rapid City, SD, December 3–5, 2013.
10. Tarr B. Cold stress in cows. Ontario Ministry of Agriculture and Food; 2007. Available at: http://www.omafra.gov.on.ca/english/livestock/beef/facts/07-001.htm. Accessed November 27, 2017.
11. American Veterinary Medical Association Policies—Disabled Livestock. Undated. Available at: https://www.avma.org/KB/Policies/Pages/Disabled-Livestock.aspx. Accessed November 27, 2017.
12. Laca A. Ranchers turn to Facebook, Twitter, to find cattle stranded by blizzard. AgWeb News 2015. Available at: https://www.agweb.com/article/ranchers-use-facebook-to-round-up-blizzard-stranded-cattle-naa-anna-lisa-laca/. Accessed November 7, 2017.
13. Hay lift aims to save snowbound Plains cattle. 2007. Available at: http://www.nbcnews.com/id/16389942/ns/weather/t/hay-lift-aims-save-snowbound-plains-cattle/#.WgYR6ohrx_A. Accessed November 27, 2017.
14. Daly R. Caring for animals when the power goes out. 2016. Available at: http://igrow.org/livestock/beef/caring-for-animals-when-the-power-goes-out/. Accessed November 27, 2017.
15. Bennett B. Colorado blizzard response, mitigation and frustration. Proceedings of the Academy of Veterinary Consultants Spring meeting. Oklahoma City, OK, April 5–7, 2007. p. 69–80.
16. Allen A. Transport tetany in ruminants. In: Kahn C, editor. Merck veterinary manual. 9th edition. Whitehouse Station (NJ): Merck & Co; 2005. p. 834–5.
17. Stewart A. Disorders of magnesium metabolism. In: Kahn C, editor. Merck veterinary manual. 9th edition. Whitehouse Station (NJ): Merck & Co; 2005. p. 812–4.
18. Anderson DE, Rings DM. Current veterinary therapy: food animal practice. 5th edition. St Louis (MO): Saunders; 2009. p. 346–60.
19. Butler L, Daly R, Wright C. Cold stress and newborn calves. 2012. Available at: https://igrow.org/up/resources/02-2001-2013.pdf. Accessed November 27, 2017.
20. Daly R. Frostbite in newborn calves. 2016. Available at: http://igrow.org/livestock/beef/frostbite-in-newborn-calves/. Accessed November 27, 2017.

# Management of Confined Cattle in Blizzard Conditions

David B. Sjeklocha, DVM

## KEYWORDS

- Blizzard • Storm • Snow • Bedding • Welfare • Water • Feed • Comfort

## KEY POINTS

- Severe winter weather is mentally and physically stressful for livestock and people.
- Preparation and understanding how to prioritize tasks are essential to minimizing the effects of the storm and allowing the feedyard to get back to a more normal routine.
- Preparation and prioritization of tasks can provide substantial benefit to the recovery effort.

## INTRODUCTION

Severe winter weather can result in extreme stress and high death loss. In most cases, these storms are predicted a few days ahead of time, so feedyards have some time to prepare. Having plans established for preparation and response to the storm after it has arrived is imperative in minimizing these issues. Veterinarians and feedyard management teams must develop these plans to make sure workers understand the priorities in regard to animal care after the storm has arrived.

## PREPARATION
### Insurance

If the cattle in the feedyard are insured against weather disasters, the veterinarian should consult with the management group and the insurance provider to determine what will be expected of him or her. In most instances, there is a set value placed on the cattle, and, of course, there is a deductible amount that must be met. The insurer will require the veterinarian to conduct necropsies on a percentage of the storm-related mortalities (usually in the range of 10%–20%), if there is a claim to be made. The veterinarian should also review the forms that the insurer will provide to document the necropsies.

The author has nothing to disclose.
Animal Health and Welfare, Cattle Empire LLC, Satanta, KS 67870, USA
*E-mail address:* drdave@cattle-empire.net

### Equipment

Feedtrucks, loaders, tractors, skid steers, bedding equipment, electric generators, etc., should all be full of fuel, engine oil checked, antifreeze checked, hydraulic reservoirs full and tire pressure checked. Batteries in all equipment should also be checked and replaced if they are weak. If severe cold is expected with the storm, all engines with block heaters should be plugged in. There should be enough fuel on hand to run all the necessary equipment for at least 5 days. Since generators are used infrequently, the fuel in their tanks may not be very fresh. If there is any question about the quality of fuel in the generator fuel tanks, the fuel should be disposed of properly and fresh fuel added back to the tanks. Make sure generators are in running condition and easily accessible. Mount snow removal blades and bunk cleaners on tractors before the storm arrives so they are immediately ready for service. Euthanasia equipment and supplies must also be ready for use. Depending on the severity of the storm and the feedyard population size, the number of animals that require euthanasia may be in the hundreds.

### Cattle Comfort

A cold, wet, driven snow will induce extraordinary stress on cattle. Feedyards can anticipate this and prepare for cattle comfort ahead of time. All pens should be cleaned thoroughly in late summer or early fall, if possible, to allow for solid footing in the case of heavy melting snow, and to also allow for tractors to operate in the pens to remove snow or provide bedding. Just prior to the storm, bales of bedding can be strategically distributed throughout the yard where they are needed most (prioritizing cattle risk will be discussed later). Windbreaks can be of value, but they must be constructed correctly. A solid windbreak can result in the wind swirling downward as it passes over the top of the windbreak, thus dropping snow on the downwind side of the windbreak. Research has shown that the most effective windbreak is 75% to 80% solid (20%–25% porous). This allows for some air to flow or "leak" through. This air that "leaks" through prevents much of the downdrafting and swirling that occurs with a solid wood fence.[1] A negative aspect of windbreak fences is that they are usually permanent structures, which may be a problem in the warmer months when more air movement is desirable.

### Workers

Consider asking a number of workers to spend the night at the feedyard as the storm moves in. Cots, sleeping bags/blankets, food, and water must be available for those workers. All employees will need to bring winter clothing – overalls, insulated boots, warm headwear, gloves, etc. Management should be prepared to provide some of these protective items in case there are workers who are in need. Depending on how much snow is expected, it may be necessary for workers to take shifts around the clock to keep roads and feed alleys open. If the storm lasts for multiple days, employees may become stranded at the feedyard, so food and water needs must be considered for this situation, as well. Feedyard cowboys will most likely not be riding pens and processing crews will not be processing cattle, so they need to be made aware that they will need to bring clothing to accommodate activities in the yard on foot.

## AFTER THE STORM HAS ARRIVED
### Prioritize

Efforts should be prioritized as follows:

1. Water supply
2. Feed
3. Cattle Comfort

Prioritization of necessities will help the feedyard crew make decisions and maintain focus. First and foremost, *water* must be available for the cattle. Tanks will need to be checked to make sure they have not frozen. Electrical power may be lost, so electric generators may be required to power wells. Second, *feed* must be delivered. This will require the feed mill being operational; snow is cleared from feed alleys, feed bunks and feed aprons; and that feed trucks and loaders are running. Again, electrical generators may be required to operate the feed mill(s). Once it is established that water and feed is or will be available, then *cattle comfort* can be addressed. If the pen floors have been well-maintained, loaders or tractors with front-mounted blades or box blades can be taken into the pens to push snow or simply make a single pass around the pen to clear an area where the cattle can lay down. Attention should also be paid to the feed apron (concrete pad behind the bunk), as all efforts to get feed to cattle will be pointless if the snow is too deep for the cattle to approach the bunk. A clean bunk pad can also serve as a relatively dry place for cattle to rest.

Ideally, bedding should be spread in the pens, as well. The cattle in the hospitals and the youngest/newest cattle in the yard (including unprocessed cattle) are *top priority* for bedding, followed by the heaviest/longest term cattle in the yard. Bedding can consist of crop residues, such as straw or corn stalks, or wood chips, if available. In some areas, wood chips are readily available and provide some advantages such as the cattle will not eat them, and they are less likely to get saturated with water than sawdust, straw or corn stalks.

### Labor Utilization

In most instances, riding pens will be a low priority. One reason for this is employee safety. Sending cowboys out on horses in slick and wet conditions could jeopardize the well-being of both the cowboys and their horses. Another reason is that the cattle will typically be huddled in groups, thus making it difficult to examine them. Processing and re-implanting will also be a low priority. Cowboys and processing crew members can be utilized in other areas that will help expedite the storm recovery effort, such as cleaning bunks, opening gates for machinery, helping to thaw out water tanks, attending to cattle in the hospitals, etc.

### Animal Welfare

Severe winter weather can result in animal suffering. Cattle tend to crowd into corners of pens as the wind-driven snow presses them to huddle up and use each other for warmth and as windbreaks. This crowding and pressing often results in cattle being crushed against fences, collapsing and being trampled by their penmates. Addressing these huddled groups is a task in which cowboys and processing crew members can be utilized. For safety reasons, at least two people should work together to go from pen to pen and break up these groups to reduce the number of cattle that are getting trampled. These workers should also take notice of any animals that may be down in the mud and unable to rise. Prognosis on these down cattle is typically grave, and a decision should quickly be made on the likelihood of their survival. All animals that are deemed unlikely to survive should be promptly euthanized, using AABP euthanasia guidelines.[2] The process of breaking up these groups and euthanizing cattle will result in physical, mental and psychological fatigue, so it would be advisable to make sure these workers are alternated frequently.

### Necropsies

If there is an insurance claim to be made, the attending veterinarian will be required to conduct necropsies on a percentage of the mortalities. Typically, the insurance provider will request a total mortality count early in the process of storm recovery. It can be very difficult to offer an accurate number, as there may be mortalities covered up in snow and mud. As the mortalities are hauled to the necropsy area, it is very important to lay them out in an orderly fashion, such as in rows. This is because the it may be a few days before the veterinarian can get the necropsies completed, and if the carcasses are stacked on top of each other, they may freeze together, making it more difficult to conduct the necropsies. Also, the insurer may request photos as evidence of the number of mortalities, the number of necropsies conducted, and to demonstrate some level of random selection of the carcasses for necropsy. Frozen carcasses can be very difficult to necropsy, so the veterinarian may need to be creative in his/her approach. It may be necessary to use an axe or chainsaw to open these carcasses. A cordless reciprocating saw can also be very helpful, but will require multiple batteries and electricity to charge them. This is another area where feedyard employees can be utilized, as the veterinarian will need to complete the necropsies as soon as possible. Feedyard employees can expedite this process by having the mortalities opened so the veterinarian can observe the animal for pathology and make notes for the insurance claim. Feedyard employees may not be skilled in knife sharpening, so it may be beneficial for the feedyard or the attending veterinarian to provide knives and sharpening equipment (steels or stones).

## SUMMARY

The effects of a blizzard on confined cattle can be devastating. Developing a workable plan and making sure all employees know their responsibilities are key to minimizing the effects of the storm. Preparation and prioritization of tasks can provide substantial benefit to the recovery effort.

## REFERENCES

1. "Windbreak fences," Beef cattle handbook, Iowa Beef Center BCH-10200. Available at: www.iowabeefcenter.org/bch/WindbreakFences.pdf. Accessed November 15, 2017.
2. "Practical euthanasia of cattle," AABP resources. Available at: www.aabp.org/resources/euth.pdf. Accessed November 15, 2017.

# Wildfire Response in Range Cattle

David N. Rethorst, DVM[a],*, Randall K. Spare, DVM[b], John L. Kellenberger, DVM[b]

**KEYWORDS**

• Wildfire • Disaster relief • Range cattle

**KEY POINTS**

• Assessing the welfare of surviving cattle, disposal of cattle lost in the fire, and support of the affected ranchers are the critical priorities after a wildfire.

• After a wildfire, cattle are typically sorted into 3 categories: cattle that succumbed in the fire, cattle that are beyond function (burned feet, burned udders, burned eyes, and severely singed hair), and cattle that appear to be unharmed.

• As a rule, ranchers are stewards of the resources that have been entrusted to their care, whether it is land, grass, or cattle. Although some ranchers are able to euthanize their own cattle in these situations, there are some who seek out veterinary assistance.

Wildfires in areas of the Great Plains during March of 2016 and 2017 left scars that will be seen and felt for years. The March 23, 2016, Anderson Creek fire burned nearly 400,000 acres in Barber and Comanche counties in south central Kansas and Woods county in north-central Oklahoma, killing approximately 600 head of cattle and destroying several hundred miles of fence. Although there were 16 homes burned in this fire and 25 other structures were destroyed, there was no loss of human life. At least 6 separate fires occurred on March 6, 2017, burning an estimated 1.2 million acres in southwest Kansas, the Oklahoma panhandle, and the Texas panhandle. The largest of these, the Starbuck fire, burned over 715,000 acres in Clark, Comanche, and Meade counties in Kansas, as well as in Beaver county Oklahoma. The Selman fire burned more than 47,000 acres in Harper and Woodward counties in Oklahoma and the 283 fire burned and additional 71,000 acres in Harper county Oklahoma. The Perryton fire burned 315,000 acres in Ochiltree, Lipscomb, and Hemphill counties in Texas, and the Lefors East fire burned 92,500 acres in Gray county Texas and the Dumas Complex fire burned more than 29,000 acres in Potter county Texas. Five people lost their lives in these fires, 1 in Kansas when a truck driver drove into the fire and 4 in the Texas panhandle while moving cattle out of the path of the fire. The Starbuck fire

The authors have nothing to disclose.
ª Beef Health Solutions, 13441 Anthony Drive, Wamego, KS 66547, USA; ᵇ Ashland Veterinary Center, 544 West 4th Avenue, Ashland, KS 67831, USA
* Corresponding author.
E-mail address: david.rethorst.dvm@gmail.com

Vet Clin Food Anim 34 (2018) 281–288
https://doi.org/10.1016/j.cvfa.2018.02.004
0749-0720/18/© 2018 Elsevier Inc. All rights reserved.

was responsible for the loss of nearly 4000 cows and 4000 calves, in addition to approximately 4100 miles of fence and 30 homes. The manner in which the producers and communities affected by the Starbuck fire dealt with the aftermath and recovery from this natural disaster is the focus of this article.

## THE IMMEDIATE NEED

Assessing the welfare of the surviving cattle, disposal of the cattle lost in the fire, and support of the affected ranchers were the critical priorities as the fire burned out. The plentiful, dormant grass that was available for grazing before March 6 was completely burned in the fire. Wheat pasture was available for grazing but not enough for the number of cows involved. Much of the baled forage that was to be fed before grass greenup was destroyed in the fire. Those ranches that had baled hay after the fire did not have enough to feed the entire herd.

Ranchers are a very self-sufficient group who are much more adept at helping others than accepting help while enduring hardship. Yet, in the nearly overwhelming aftermath of the Starbuck fire, the affected ranchers soon realized that they did need help. The fire was not completely out before semi-trailer truck loads of donated hay were on the road headed to the area so that the surviving cows could be fed. People were calling, asking what their boots on the ground could do to help. Others did not call, rather, just showed up asking, "What can I do?" Others donated milk replacer for the surviving calves whose mothers succumbed in the fire. A veterinarian who works for a dairy calf ranch took calves and placed them in hutches at the calf ranch so they had shelter, milk replacer, and water. In an adjoining county, 4-H groups took in calves to care for so ranchers could focus on other needs.

With all of these needs being addressed simultaneously, in addition to the need to communicate with the Kansas Department of Health and Environment on disposal of dead cows, leadership and coordination was needed. The veterinarians of Ashland Veterinary Center made the decision early, the morning after the fire, that they would act as coordinators of the relief effort, in addition to going alongside their producer clients to assist them during these extenuating circumstances; essentially becoming command central for all things related to the area livestock. One veterinarian stayed at the clinic, answering phone calls, matching hay with ranchers in need, coordinating the effort to care for the surviving calves, talking to the Federal Emergency Management Agency, and directing assisting veterinarians to ranches who needed help assessing the aftermath. Another veterinarian from the clinic focused on assisting clients most affected by the fire, while others filled in as necessary. Later in the week after the fire, many of the command central duties were assigned to volunteers in the community to spread out the work load. These tasks included managing monetary donations, managing donations of fencing supplies, coordination of housing for volunteers, and providing meals for volunteers.

## ASSESSMENT, EUTHANASIA, AND DISPOSAL

Three categories of cattle existed after the fire. First and most obvious were the cattle that succumbed in the fire that needed to be documented for insurance purposes or US Department of Agriculture (USDA) Livestock Indemnity Program (LIP) payments and then disposed of in a proper manner. The second group were cattle that were burned beyond function. This group included cows with burned feet, burned udders, burned eyes, and severely singed hair (**Figs. 1–6**). The top priority was to humanely euthanize these cows and dispose of them. The third group were cows that appeared to be unharmed.

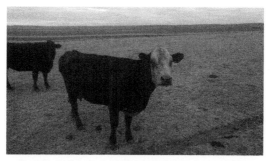

**Fig. 1.** Group 2 cow after fire. Note burned eyes and singed hair. Feet and udder were also burned on this cow. (*Courtesy of* David Rethorst, DVM, Beef Health Solutions, Wamego, KS.)

As a rule, ranchers are stewards of the resources that have been entrusted to their care, whether it be land, grass, or cattle. They knew there were cows that required feed and calves to be dealt with but their primary objective after the fire was to find those cows that needed to be humanely euthanized. These cows typically had severely burned feet and udders. Many of their eyes were burned and hair coats singed, and there were burns over much of their bodies. Some ranchers were able to euthanize these cows themselves, whereas others sought veterinary assistance because they could not bring themselves to euthanize cows they had raised and taken care of for several years. Documentation of the deaths of these cows and the cows that died during the fire was required for insurance purposes or the LIP. Photographs, head counts, and third-party verification provided this documentation.

After the severely burned cows had been humanely euthanized, the focus turned to the surviving cows. This group of cows initially appeared normal after the fire. Within a matter of a few days, however, it became apparent that a good percentage of these cows had enough heat damage to the coronary band that there was separation of the coronary band and/or they had udder damage. Based on experiences gained in the aftermath of the 2016 Anderson Creek fire, it was generally accepted that these cows would not be productive going forward. An issue with LIP that became apparent when dealing with this disaster is the psychological stress that the program creates as producers and veterinarians deal with the financial and animal welfare issues associated with documenting the dead animals, euthanizing suffering animals, and deciding

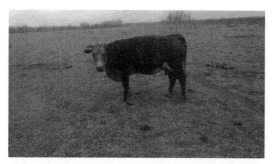

**Fig. 2.** Group 2 cow after fire. Note burned eyes and udder, as well as singed hair. Feet were also burned on this cow. (*Courtesy of* David Rethorst, DVM, Beef Health Solutions, Wamego, KS.)

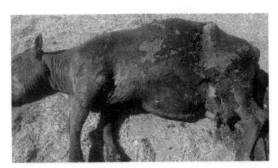

**Fig. 3.** Group 2 cow after euthanasia. Note severely burned eyes, skin, and udder. (*Courtesy of* David Rethorst, DVM, Beef Health Solutions, Wamego, KS.)

which animals could go into the food chain rather than being euthanized. These ranchers do not want to see their animals suffer, so making the decision to put down animals that lived through the fire but had severely burned feet, udders, or eyes, was not a difficult decision. The problem was with the cows that were burned enough that they would not be productive for the ranch in future years, yet could potentially go into the food chain. Thought had to be given to the question of whether the cows were suffering too much to put them on a truck to the packing plant. Another consideration was what would happen if they were condemned at the packing plant. In order for cows to be eligible for the indemnity, they had to succumb during the fire or be euthanized on the ranch. Cows condemned at the packing plant were not eligible for indemnity; if they had been euthanized on the ranch, they would have been eligible for indemnity. Cows that passed inspection at the plant did not, in most cases, bring as much money as was being paid for indemnity. Again, if these cows had been euthanized on the ranch, they would be eligible for full indemnity. However, these ranchers wanted these cows to be used for a productive purpose, so they sent them to the packing plant. Perhaps these cows should be eligible for the difference between market price at the packing plant and the indemnity price.

A low percentage of the cows involved in this fire were covered by mortality insurance due to the high cost of this insurance and the low likelihood of an event that would cause the death of this many cows. If the cows were insured, there was more latitude in the cows that could be sent to slaughter because insurance would pay the full insured value on cows that did not pass harvest inspection, as well as

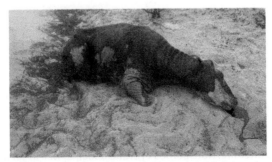

**Fig. 4.** Group 2 cow after euthanasia. Note singed hair, severely burned eyes and skin. (*Courtesy of* David Rethorst, DVM, Beef Health Solutions, Wamego, KS.)

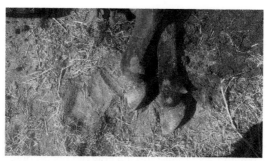

**Fig. 5.** Feet of **Fig. 3** cow. Note separation of coronary band. (*Courtesy of* David Rethorst, DVM, Beef Health Solutions, Wamego, KS.)

the difference between slaughter value and insured value of the cows. In certain instances, it seemed as if the assessing veterinarian was making major financial decisions for these ranchers. As stewards of the land, the grass, and the cows, ranchers do not like to see any of these resources wasted. They are used to creating value by managing resources and reducing waste. Seeing cows put down that would have normally gone into the food supply challenged the thinking of these stewards.

A variety of firearms were used in the euthanasia process. Pistols ranging from .22 magnum to 9 mm, .357 magnum, and .45 caliber were very effective in dealing with the cows that were humanely euthanized immediately after the fire. Due to their inability to move quickly because of burned coronary bands and their inability to see well because of burned eyes, these cows could be euthanized at very close range. The .22 magnum proved very effective on these cows and there certainly less noise associated with this firearm than there was with the higher caliber pistols. Hollow point or personal protection type ammunition proved to be inconsistent even at close range. The landmarks described in Beef Quality Assurance training proved effective if the shooters were knowledgeable of the landmarks and the firearm was side-to-side perpendicular to the cow's skull.[1]

Rifles were the firearm of choice for the cows that initially appeared normal but had to be euthanized several days later because these cows could see well and move well enough that it was difficult to get close enough to them to use a pistol. A wide range of rifles were found to be effective at the ranges shooters were working from, including

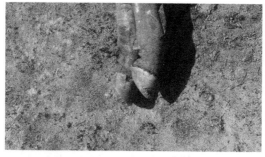

**Fig. 6.** Feet of group 2 cow after euthanasia. Note separation of coronary band on foot on the right and hoof wall coming off of coffin bone on leg on the left. (*Courtesy of* David Rethorst, DVM, Beef Health Solutions, Wamego, KS.)

.22 rifles with solid point long rifle rounds, .22 magnum rifles with solid point rounds, and various high-power rifles. Scoped, high power rifles were found to be less than optimally effective at the range at which shooters were working because these rifles were sighted in at distances of several hundred yards. Again, critical to this process is the ability to consistently and effectively hit the external landmarks at the proper angles so that the brainstem is destroyed.

Consideration should be given to other factors, such as that use of a scope limits the peripheral vison of the shooter creating possible human safety concerns, considering the number of people that are involved in situation such as this. Many of the cattle that required euthanasia were in pastures or large traps where there was no fence. If distances were not estimated accurately and the cow did not go down, they would take off and it was hard to get another shot on the cow. Other cows would charge the shooter if the shot was missed.

Observation of the psychological impact of the euthanasia process on the remaining cows was interesting. In unconfined situations, the remaining cows would generally run as a cow was put down. On some occasions, one of the remaining cows would charge the shooter as her herd-mate went down. In a confined setting, some the remaining cows would turn their tails to the shooter after a few cows had been put down. This makes a good case for sedation of the cattle, if at all possible, before euthanizing a group of cows by gunshot. Sedation would alleviate the anxiety that was observed in these cows, as well as allow the use of a small caliber firearm, which would reduce the psychological stress on the humans involved in the process.

It became very apparent in the aftermath of this fire that a protocol for a chemical euthanasia agent that could be fed to cattle should be developed. A chemical agent that would cause a rapid humane death would reduce anxiety in livestock and humans alike. This is especially true if a foreign animal disease outbreak should ever occur in this country and thousands of cattle need to be euthanized in a very short order. The use of cyanide or nitrate has been suggested.

Because of the respect the involved ranchers have for their livestock, it was imperative that the dead cows were buried as soon as possible. Through timely and open communication with the Kansas Department of Health and Environment, cooperation was forthcoming in the disposal of the animals destroyed in the fire as well as those euthanized. The recommended guidelines were to dig the burial pits on high ground, place no more than 100 cows per pit, and make sure there was at least 3 feet of dirt placed on top of the buried cows. No permit was required for the burial of these cows. Coordination with 800-DIG-SAFE provided safe locations for the burial pits. Global positioning system (GPS) coordinates were recorded for many of the pits.

## DISASTER RELIEF AND REBUILDING

The USDA Farm Service Agency (FSA) has indemnity programs to assist producers affected by disasters such as this.[2] These programs are deficient when dealing with the scope of loss that occurs on large production systems in such disasters.

The National Cattlemen's Beef Association's *Beef Industry Statistics* reports that the average cow herd size in the United States is 40 cows, yet the average cow herd size in the region affected by this fire is several times that.[3] Some ranches have cow herds numbering 500 to 1000. There are ranches in the fire area that lost 600 or more cows, in addition to newborn calves and replacement stock. The 2017 LIP payment of $1038.73 per cow is based on 75% of average fair market value of the livestock as determined by the USDA.[2] A facet of the LIP that created challenges for these ranchers is the clause that states "no person or legal entity, excluding a joint venture or general partnership, may receive directly or indirectly, more than $125,000 total in payments under the Livestock Forage Disaster Program, Emergency Assistance for Livestock, Honeybees and Farm-Raised Fish Program and LIP combined per program year."[2] Dividing the $125,000 cap by the per-cow payment of $1038.73 reveals that ranchers got paid for, at most, 120 cows. If they lost 600 cows, as was the case for several ranchers, the LIP payment comes up woefully short of truly helping these ranchers. If the cows were owned by a general partnership, each partner was eligible for a full indemnity payment; however, if the same number of cows was owned by a family corporation, eligibility was limited to 1 indemnity payment. This payment cap was very inadequate for some ranchers affected by this fire because there are ranches that lost 200 to 700 cows, in addition to calves and replacement stock. Legislation has been introduced as a result of the aftermath of the Starbuck fire that will, it is hoped, alleviate the problems with LIP that became apparent after the Starbuck fire, in future natural disasters.

The Emergency Conservation Program (ECP) administered by FSA provides cost-share funds to rebuild the hundreds of miles of fence that were destroyed in this fire.[4] This cost share pays 75% of the cost to rebuild the fence up to a cap of $200,000.[4] Again, in some instances, this program does not adequately address the needs in this area because of the size of the ranches involved. For example, if a ranch is running 600 cows at a stocking rate of 20 acres per cow on a year-round basis, it will take 12,000 acres (19 sections) to run the cows. Ten miles of fence will be required to fence 3 contiguous sections at a rate of $10,000 per mile of fence for materials and labor. This per-section cost of $33,333 means it will require $633,327 to fence the 19 sections, which is $433,327 higher than the cap.

It is understood that there must be rules anytime FSA is providing disaster relief. However, the rules that accompany the ECP fence program are a burden in and of themselves. If a portion of the fence is changed in any way, that portion of the fence is not eligible for the program. If a knob is leveled to make replacing the fence easier or a small washout is filled in as the fence is rebuilt, the fence is changed enough that it is not eligible for the program. A double-H brace is required each one-quarter mile if there is not a gate or other structure in that one-quarter mile. This requirement is over and above generally accepted fencing practices in the area and significantly adds to the cost of replacing the fence, not only material cost but also time and labor costs.

The truly amazing thing seen in the relief and recovery effort following this disaster was the outpouring of love and caring from the agricultural community nationwide. Hundreds of bales of hay were donated and hauled to the area for the affected ranchers. Much of this hay was unloaded at hay depots that had been established near the local feed mill and at an area ranch so that the ranchers could pick up hay as they needed it. Other donated hay was hauled directly to area ranches by those donating it. Fencing materials arrived by the truck and trailer load, again donated by fellow farmers and ranchers in surrounding states. Monetary donations poured into the Ashland Foundation and the Kansas Livestock Association Foundation to be distributed to the area ranchers. At auction markets in the region, roll-over auctions were held at which an animal was sold numerous times with the money being donated to the relief efforts. In some instances, heifers were donated to some of the more severely affected ranchers.

## THE PSYCHOLOGICAL EFFECT

The psychological stress created in those people associated with the euthanasia process is not to be taken lightly. This stress occurs for several reasons, including the raw emotions of euthanizing genetic stock that ranchers have spent their lifetimes developing; the number of animals requiring euthanasia; the noise level created when using firearms to euthanize animals, especially a large group of animals; and the length of time that this process requires. Field officers from the Kansas Department of Wildlife, Parks, and Tourism assisted in the euthanasia process, which relieved a portion of the emotional stress in the producers and veterinarians involved in this process.

A comment heard numerous times in the week after the fire was, "The first gunshot was the easiest," because the first cow that a person euthanized was the easiest to put down and as each successive cow was euthanized psychological stress mounted. Some ranchers chose to euthanize their own cows, feeling they owed it to their cows because the cows provided them a living, whereas other ranchers could not bring themselves to euthanize their own cows and needed assistance in performing this task. Regardless of who was performing the euthanasia, this stress was not to be taken lightly. Having numerous people who understood the landmarks used for euthanasia and were competent with firearms helped distribute this stress.

In the weeks and months following this disaster, there was concern that those heavily affected by the fire would suffer from posttraumatic stress disorder. Again, the love and caring of friends, neighbors, and the agricultural community of the state and nation helped these ranchers get through this psychological stress. Phone calls, a quick note, or a timely visit showed these ranchers that people were thinking about them and cared about them, which helped tremendously.

## SUMMARY

Conceptualization has been defined as the ability to take multiple, ambiguous, seemingly disconnected circumstances and order the chaos into a sensible strategy to solve a problem. This is a skill that is inherent.[5] It cannot be taught, yet it can be improved on. It is a skill that is prevalent in progressive rural veterinarians and the producers that they serve. Because of the relationships that these veterinarians have with the producers they serve, they are able to use their conceptualization skills to provide leadership when disasters such as the Starbuck Fire occur. These working relationships cannot be replaced by government intervention in disasters. Because of the caring attitude that veterinarians have for their clientele and the trust that the clients have in their veterinarians, assistance from Federal Emergency Management Agency was not necessary. It is about integrity first, service above self, and excellence in service provided.

## REFERENCES

1. Beef Quality Assurance–Supplemental Guidelines 2014. Available at: www.bqa.org.
2. Livestock Indemnity Program (LIP)–United States Department of Agriculture Farm Service Agency. Available at: www.fsa.usda.gov/programs-and-services/disaster-assistance-programs/livestock-indemnity-program.
3. Beef Industry Statistics–Beef USA. Available at: www.beefusa.org/beef industrystatistics.aspx.
4. Emergency Conservation Program (ECP)–United States Department of Agriculture Farm Service Agency. Available at: www.fsa.usda.gov/programs-and-services/conservation-programs/emergency-conservation-program.
5. Barringer L. Kansas State University Upson Lecture Series. 2017.

# Preparation and Response to Truck Accidents on Highways Involving Cattle

Lisa Pederson, M.Agr[a],*, Jerry Yates, BS[b], Audry Wieman, DVM[c]

## KEYWORDS

- Cattle transportation • Emergency response • Standard operating procedures
- Accidents • Humane euthanasia

## KEY POINTS

- Annually, in the United States, more than 50 million head of cattle are transported. The majority are transported via semitrailer.
- As the number of livestock transported via motor vehicle has increased, so has the number of accidents involving livestock transport. Most livestock transport accidents in the United States involved semitrailers carrying cattle.
- Before the Bovine Emergency Response Program, no standard operating procedures existed for accidents involving livestock transport in the United States.
- The Bovine Emergency Response Plan provides a framework for veterinarians, emergency responders, and law enforcement to better address accidents involving cattle transport.
- The plan includes standardized procedures and materials for veterinarians, dispatchers, and first responders in the areas of call assessment, scene arrival and evaluation, site containment and security, extraction of cattle from the trailer, relocation of cattle involved in the accident, convalescence, mortality disposal, righting of the transport vehicle, humane euthanasia, and debriefing.

## INTRODUCTION

Annually, more than 50 million head of domestic and imported cattle and calves are marketed and transported for breeding, feeding, and slaughter in the United States. Nearly all of these cattle are transported via trucks and semitrailers known as pots (**Fig. 1**).

According to a 2007 news article, in a 7-year period, more than 400 livestock transport accidents were reported in the United States and Canada. Of these accidents,

The authors have nothing to disclose.
[a] North Dakota State University Extension, Central Grasslands Research Extension Center, 4824 48th Avenue SE, Streeter, ND 58483, USA; [b] Reymann Memorial Farms, West Virginia University Davis College of Agriculture, Natural Resources and Design, 1695 State Route 259 North, Wardensville, WV 26851, USA; [c] Ridgeline Vet Services, LLC, 89493 509 Avenue, Lynch, NE 68746, USA
* Corresponding author.
*E-mail address:* Lisa.Pederson@ndsu.edu

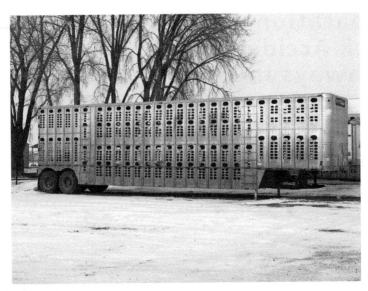

**Fig. 1.** A cattle pot.

56% involved cattle trucks. Of the 169 documented cattle truck accidents, 23% involved trucks hauling finished cattle to slaughter and 70% involved the transport of feeders and calves. Most of the accidents occurred in October, followed by November, August, April, and May. Despite the time of year, only 1% of the reports identify weather as a cause of the accident.[1,2] The increase in accidents in these months coincides with the increases in movement of feeder cattle from farms and ranches through marketing facilities such as livestock auction markets to feedlot operations.

Animal health authorities, law enforcement, livestock industries, first responders, and livestock transport industries have long identified a need for standard operating procedures to address cattle transportation accidents. In 2011, the Bovine Emergency Response Program (BERP) was developed to address this need. The objectives of the Bovine Emergency Response Plan are: (1) to develop a framework that local veterinarians, law enforcement, first responders, and emergency management can use to more appropriately address accidents involving cattle transport vehicles. This framework is rigid enough to cover all of the critically needed areas but flexible enough to fit the needs of local municipalities; (2) to identify further educational materials and curriculum related to the project; and (3) to identify future funding needs related to the development and sustainability of the Bovine Emergency Response Plan and its associated educational materials and program. This article discusses the components of the BERP and how veterinarians can be involved in preparing for and responding to truck accidents involving cattle.

## THE VETERINARIAN'S ROLE IN TRUCK ACCIDENTS ON HIGHWAYS

Veterinarians should be involved in developing the details of the BERP with their local first responders. Although the veterinarian plays many vital roles in the entire process, primary among them is providing expertise and oversight in the evaluation and care of the animals involved in the accident. Veterinarians will also benefit from being engaged in the entire process and developing relationships with first responders. The reciprocal is true for emergency management teams. Even in rural America, societal changes have resulted in less knowledge of animal behavior and overall situational awareness. A shared vision ensures the appropriate personnel are trained and contacted at the right time during an emergency, setting in motion a cascade of events that culminates in a successful outcome. The only way that happens is to "Build your team before you get on scene"!

## PREPAREDNESS

In order to successfully mitigate one of these accidents, advanced preparation is critical. A plan should be developed and then used to further develop and complete training for key individuals involved. The plan should also be shared with county emergency management.

An "Emergency Contact Sheet" and "Dispatcher Decision Tree" should be developed before incident (Appendices 1 and 2). Essential personnel should be identified in preplanning exercises. Safety and security require that only essential and trained personnel be granted access to the scene. Each responder should develop a list of items needed and determine the best way to have quick and easy access.

Containment plans should include a list of local entities (individuals and businesses) that can quickly and adeptly provide livestock-handling equipment needed to "build" a containment facility as well as instructions on how to erect containment facilities in many different accident scenarios.

Relocation plans for surviving livestock should be developed before an emergency. These entities should be included in the Emergency Contact Sheet (see Appendix 1). All relocation facilities must have at minimum basic animal-handling equipment available for treatment of injured animals, the ability to isolate the relocated animals from existing herds and other new arrivals, and the ability to feed stressed animals (long-stem hay, fresh water). The following type of facilities may meet the criteria for a relocation facility:

- Fairgrounds or other livestock show event locations with facilities (arenas)
- Auction markets, buying stations
- Cattle operations (feed yards, backgrounders, cow/calf operations)

Develop relationships with the local agricultural community to ensure immediate access to smaller livestock trailers, portable corral-type panels and other livestock fencing-related materials, and especially steel posts and a driving aid. Community members agreeing to provide these necessary items should be detailed on the Emergency Contact Sheet (see Appendix 1).

### *Preparedness Checklist*

- Complete "Emergency Contact Sheet" (see Appendix 1) Dispatcher Decision Tree (see later discussion)
- Share BERP and all associated documentation with the appropriate responders and authorities
- Conduct training with first responders and those on "Emergency Contact Sheet" annually at the minimum
- Inclusion of Bovine (Livestock) Emergency Response Plan into the County Emergency Plan
- Development of and training on the containment plans
- Assembly of "tool kit" for first responders and veterinarians
  - Pens and pencils
  - Clipboard or notebook
  - Paper
  - The Animal Transport Incident Assessment Form

o Copy of Emergency Contact List, relocation plans, mortality disposal plan
o Record-keeping forms for mortalities and morbidities, treatment, and euthanasia records
o Flashlight
o Rope halter
o Rope
o Smooth wire
o Wire cutters
o Livestock paint chalk/stick
o Pole syringe and anesthetic for dealing with fractious animals inside a trailer
o Euthanasia tool and required ammunition or charge, and pithing rod if using a captive bolt stun (please see Jan K. Shearer and colleagues' article, "Humane Euthanasia and Carcass Disposal," in this issue).
o Hot shot and other driving aids
o Sharp knives
o Chains strong enough to assist in morality removal, securing fences, and so forth
o A small tool kit, including wire cutters, hammer, fencing staples, and some chain quick repair links with threaded couplers

## RESPONSE
### Dispatcher Decision Tree

The Dispatcher Decision Tree has been developed to help prepare first responders for their response to the livestock transportation incident. It is designed to ask the incident reporting party a scripted set of questions that will set in motion a smoother, safer, and more efficient response. Veterinarians' names and contact information should be included in the "Emergency Contact Sheet" (see Appendix 1), and they should be among the first called in the incident response.

When the call comes into the dispatch center, the dispatcher will ask the following:

- Location, number calling from, name of person calling, type of emergency
- If animals are involved in the accident
  o No, continue to standard accident dispatcher decision tree
  o Yes, continue to Bovine Emergency Response Dispatcher Decision Tree

Bovine Emergency Response Dispatcher Decision Tree

- Type of incident
  o Animal versus vehicle (hitting deer, cow, other animal)
    ▪ If this type of incident, continue to specific decision tree for collisions
  o Vehicle versus vehicle hauling livestock
  o Single vehicle hauling livestock
- Type or types of vehicles involved
  o Pickup and stock trailer
  o Truck and semitrailer
- Are there livestock/animals loose on the scene?
- What types of livestock or animals are involved?
- Is fire involved?
- Are hazardous chemicals involved?
- Are the vehicle or vehicles
  o Upright and on their wheels
  o Rolled

  - ■ To the left
  - ■ To the right
  - o Jackknifed

Dispatcher then reports the above available information to the responding law enforcement and first responders and initiates the call list from the Emergency Contact Sheet.

Once first responders are dispatched, owners/managers of relocation facilities need to be alerted that surviving livestock may be relocated to their operation when the dispatcher takes the initial call.

### Emergency Response on Arrival

### Secure perimeter

- Establish a scene perimeter. Make the perimeter far larger than needed to allow for space to work and to buffer livestock from stressful sights (flashing lights) and sounds (sirens, horns, radios, and so forth). Safety and security require that only essential and trained personnel be granted access to the scene.
  - o Approach scene involving animals as calmly and quietly as possible. Do not immediately attempt to get the animals up or moving; do not stick lights, limbs, or objects inside the trailer before being ready for extraction. Do not extract animals from the trailer until a containment structure is in place. Livestock extraction before having a containment structure erected almost always results in preventable injuries to humans and livestock, secondary vehicular accidents, and/or death.
  - o Limit the use of sirens, horns, and other loud noises, including loud talking, shouting, bullhorns, and radios. Cell phones and text messaging may be the most effective way to communicate between responders while minimizing noise stress to animals.
  - o Limit the use of flashing lights, especially at night.
  - o Limit the use of reflective gear at night. It causes confusion in already agitated livestock.
  - o Be prepared for potential conflict about the amount of time the road should safely be closed versus the pressures to get the road open. Prolonged closures (>8 hours) are often common depending on the severity of the accident.

### Scene safety

- Secure the vehicles involved.
- Take actions to deal with any life-threatening situations. *Don't become another victim!*
  - o Fire
  - o Traffic
  - o Livestock that are loose on the scene and aggressive livestock
  - o Water
  - o Environmental conditions on location (ice, snow, rain, and so forth)

### Assess scene

- If driver is coherent
  - o Is he or she able to assist with the accident assessment?
  - o Ask him or her for the "bill of lading." Use the bill of lading to develop the "Animal Transport Incident Assessment" (see Appendix 2). Items to identify from the bill of lading include the following:
    - ■ Type and number of livestock
    - ■ Where load originated

- Where load was to be off-loaded
- Who owns the livestock being hauled
- Who is the insurer
- Are any animals involved individually insured (likely animals that are valued higher than market value)
- Assess other scene-specific conditions, such as physical limitations and/or potential onsite assets, such as roadway fencing, alleys, and other vehicles and livestock trailers.

### Assess animal situation

- Are any animals loose from the trailer involved in the accident?
  - Yes
    - Make every attempt to secure these animals for human safety as well as traffic safety.
    - Are loose animals off the highway, away from the scene, in a fenced, secure area (pasture, farmyard, field,and so forth)?
      - Yes
        - Leave them where they are.
      - No
        - Make every attempt to have loose animals secured away from the accident. Options for securing these animals include the following:
          - In a fenced pasture or farm ground
          - In an erected containment operation
- Do any of these animals need to be euthanized?
  - Yes
    - Contain "sound" loose animals.
    - Conduct euthanasia following euthanasia guide.
  - No
    - Contain "sound" loose animals.
- Continue with scene evaluation.

### Notes

Well-intended individuals who are not qualified or trained in livestock accident response will want to be involved. Examples of ideal tasks for these individuals (depending on ability) are as follows: carrying panels, affixing tarps and barriers, assisting with keeping records (ie, Animal Transport Incident Assessment), counting livestock, keeping gates closed, and similar tasks.

The information regarding the orientation of the vehicle is important because it will generally determine how first responders approach removing livestock from the trailer.

Remember the animals involved in the accident have been subjected to much additional stress, are scared, are often injured, and may react with different actions than described in the Classes of Cattle (Appendix 3). Never trust any animal. They are not capable of understanding you are only here to help! Low-stress techniques and manipulation of the fight or flight mechanism are not feasible at this point.

It is good to have a "scribe" with you to take notes and complete the Animal Transport Incident Assessment (see Appendix 2).

### Evaluate animal situation

- Understand stock type, ownership, management control, and insurance implications.

- Determine the classes of cattle with which you are dealing. Many trailers can have mixed classes of livestock on the same load (for example, cows, calves and bulls, dairy cows, and beef cows).
- Begin to build a comprehensive account of all animals encountered, including uninjured, mortality (dead animals), morbidity (sick animals), and any other relevant information pertaining to animal movement (for example, reports of animals far from scene, roaming, unaccounted for, or discrepancies in animals present vs bill of lading or verbal reports from driver). Including this information in the Animal Transport Incident Assessment (see Appendix 2) is critical.
  - Special circumstances and conditions can apply to international-origin animals, specific pathogen-free, or other "health-certified" or condemned animals.
  - Other extenuating circumstances too numerous to mention could apply, so the better the initial record, the better the postincident response documentation will be. The better the documentation, the more likely attending veterinarians and other professionals will be compensated for their professional services.

### Develop further action plans

**Security** Once the initial perimeter is secured, the scene must be further protected to maintain safety for the first responders involved, the public, and the livestock. Responders will have to develop a controlled area to keep the livestock "contained" within the accident scene, and to keep the public, including the news media, away from the accident scene.

A public information officer (PIO) should be designated for these types of incidents before having to respond to a vehicular incident involving livestock. The PIO is the only entity authorized to release information to the news media and the public during and after the accident. The PIO and their contact information should be listed in the "Emergency Contact List" (see Appendix 1).

Visual observation should be obscured from the public and news media. Tarps, plywood, and uninvolved vehicles are all items that can be used to obscure visual observation from the general public and the news media. All items should be securely affixed to fences, panels, and so forth to avoid potential injury to first responders and livestock. Furthermore, the noise of flapping from items like tarps can further excite already scared livestock.

Before any animals are extricated from the trailer, a containment structure must be put in place. In several documented cases, emergency responders or bystanders have been severely injured or killed because this critical step was not enacted.

### Containment and animal handling

- Assess demeanor of animals. First responders should understand what scared, agitated, and aggressive cattle look like. The position of the head and tail provide good clues on the demeanor of cattle (**Figs. 2** and **3**). Low-stress cattle handling tips may not work in these situations.
- Assess number of animals involved
  - Use **Figs. 4** and **5** to estimate lengths of common livestock trailers and semi-trailers and the number of cattle hauled in them.
- Contain loose animals.
  - These animals likely will be scared and may be aggressive.
  - Use natural containment conditions if present (pasture, street alley, and so forth).
  - Animals found on scene outside the vehicle that meet euthanasia criteria should be dealt with immediately. Please see Jan K. Shearer and colleagues'

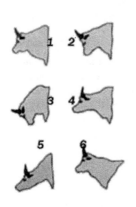

1 Neutral position

2 Slightly antagonistic position

3 Highly antagonistic position

4 Confident approach

5 Submissive approach

6 Alert before flight position

Fig. 2. Head positions of different dispositions of cattle.

article, "Humane Euthanasia and Carcass Disposal," in this issue for guidance on euthanasia.

o Livestock injured but deemed recoverable need to be contained as soon as feasible (get outside animals captured before starting inside trailer rescue and recovery).

 ■ Remember, domestic farm animals have a herding instinct and will attempt to return to the herd or find groups of animals to join. The desire to return to where they came from (accident scene/truck) is strong in most farm animal species.

 ■ Cautionary note: a situation may arise in which moving livestock is impossible without risking the health and safety of you or other personnel at the scene. Be prepared for such a situation. If safe, competent handling and/ or sedation are not options, destroying the animals is more prudent than risking injury or death to humans.

 ■ Periodically, animals will develop an aggressive or "fighting" behavioral response when stressed via an accident. Immediate and lethal action is an appropriate means to deal with these animals if they pose a danger to

1 Grazing or walking

2 Cold, ill or frightened

3 Threatening, curiosity or sexual excitement

4 Galloping

5 Kicking or playing

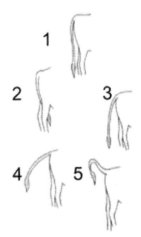

Fig. 3. Tail positions of different dispositions of cattle.

| Recommended maximum number of cattle[a] for trailers of different lengths[b]. | | | | | | | | | [a] This chart represents the maximum number of polled/dehorned cattle for trailers of different lengths; when hauling horned/tipped cattle reduced the number of cattle by 5%. |
|---|---|---|---|---|---|---|---|---|---|
| **Cattle weight, Lbs** | | | | | | | | | |
| Trailer size | 400 | 600 | 800 | 1000 | 1200 | 1400 | 1600 | Total Wt.[c] | [b] The number of cattle loaded during hot conditions should be reduced. |
| (Inside Dimension) | | | **Number of head** | | | | | | [c] The maximum weight of cattle for each trailer size with these calculations. Do not exceed the Gross Vehicle Weight Rating for your truck and stock trailer. |
| 16 ft x 6 ft | 18 | 12 | 9 | 7 | 6 | 5 | 5 | <7400 | |
| 18 ft x 6 ft | 21 | 14 | 10 | 8 | 7 | 6 | 5 | <8400 | |
| 20 ft x 6 ft | 23 | 15 | 12 | 9 | 8 | 7 | 6 | <9300 | |
| 24 ft x 6 ft | 28 | 18 | 14 | 11 | 9 | 8 | 7 | <11100 | |
| 20 ft x 7 ft | 27 | 18 | 13 | 11 | 9 | 8 | 7 | <10800 | |
| 24 ft x 7 ft | 32 | 22 | 16 | 13 | 11 | 9 | 8 | <13000 | |
| 32 ft x 7 ft | 43 | 29 | 22 | 17 | 14 | 12 | 11 | <17300 | |

Beef Quality Assurance    BEEF ✓    Funded by The Beef Checkoff

**Fig. 4.** Lengths of stock trailers and estimated number of cattle. (*Courtesy of* Jim Turner, Dee Griffin, Clyde Lane, Ronald Gill, 2008, Stock trailer transportation of cattle: Transporting the BQA way. National Beef Quality Assurance Program; with permission.)

### 48 ft – 50,000 lb Gross – Fat Cattle

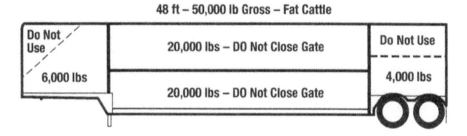

### 53 ft – 55,000 lb Gross – Feeder Cattle Lighter Than 700 lbs

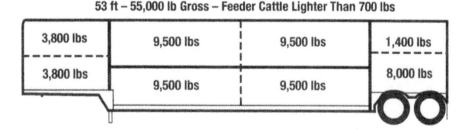

### 53 ft – 55,000 lb Gross – Fat Cattle

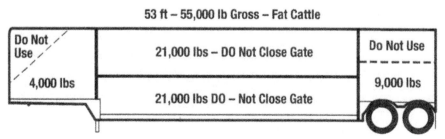

**Fig. 5.** Common lengths of semitrailers used for hauling cattle.

human safety. If used, a large-caliber rifle should be used. Considering distance and other conditions; if a shot is taken, aim for the chest, head, or neck.

- Design containment facility.
  - Evaluate the area to determine what assets are available to use as a secured, stable barrier.
    - Roadside fences
    - Uninvolved stock trailers
    - The sides or top of the involved trailer
      - Stock trailers are often between 9 and 30 feet in length
      - Semitrailers are generally between 40 and 50 feet in length
  - Use the Animal Transport Incident Assessment Form (see Appendix 2), the bill of lading, and verbal communications with the driver, if possible, to determine the size of the containment facility needed. As well, evaluate the scene to identify physical limitations and potential onsite assets, such as roadway fencing, alleys, other vehicles, and livestock trailers.
  - Keep pen size relating to animal numbers (too large and too small) in mind. Guidelines for pen sizes (area in square feet = width × height)[3]:
    - Larger, mature cattle (800 pounds and greater): 20 square feet per animal (if 40 head are on the truck, 800 square feet of pen space would be ideal).
    - Smaller, immature cattle (800 pounds and less): 14 square feet per animal (if 100 head are on the truck, 1400 square feet of pen space would be ideal).
  - Build a fence in a zigzag pattern and remember to secure turns or angles with steel posts.
  - Secure panels in multiple locations (at a minimum, both ends and in the middle).
  - Secure panels to each other at the top and bottom!
  - If feasible, use release and containment pens that adjoin each other but are physically separated to decrease the animal's natural desire to return to the truck. This will become easier once a few animals are held in the containment pen.
    - Consider physical properties of the barriers and any limitations to effective containment (gaps between panel rails; height, especially too short; gap at bottom); consider flipping panels over in the case of pigs, goats, sheep, and smaller bovine ruminants.
  - Design the holding pens to provide smaller livestock trailers easy access to load animals for relocation.
  - Remember that other equipment will be used at the scene, so do not block their access.
  - Ensure that the relocation fleet of trucks will not encounter obstacles or environmental issues that hinder movement.
- Use humane euthanasia as needed.
- Extrication of livestock
  - Human safety always is more important than livestock safety.
  - Rescuers should avoid entering the trailer before extrication whenever possible. Entering the trailer will become a necessity at some point, but limit potential human exposure to danger.
  - Livestock that are being off-loaded from a wrecked trailer will be scared and agitated. Take all precautions to assure emergency responder safety.
  - Before any extrication occurs, a safe, secure containment facility must be in place. Failure to have a safe, secure containment facility has caused human and livestock injuries and deaths.
  - Typically, livestock will exit the trailer at a rapid pace. Making sure the containment facility is secure and stable is critical. This includes the following:

- ▪ If joining panels to the trailers, whether involved or uninvolved in the accident, use wire or chains
- ▪ Tie corral panels to posts driven into the ground with wire or chains on the top and bottom of each panel.
- ○ Make every effort to avoid off-loading livestock onto pavement or concrete. If this is the only option, cover the roadway with sand or soil. Livestock slip on paved/concrete road surfaces. When livestock slip, they become scared, more agitated, and more dangerous to humans and often become injured or more severely injured.
- ○ If livestock need to cross the lines on a highway, cover the lines with sand or soil. Livestock typically will balk and not cross lines on a highway.
- ○ Use of animal driving aids (sticks, paddles, and so forth) can be beneficial, but limit their use and be prudent and judicious when deciding to use them.
- ○ Determine the best location to open the trailer. This will be dependent on how the trailer lies (rolled to left or right, upright, hazards on the scene, other).
  - ▪ If a trailer is on its side, extraction is easiest through the roof and rear gate. The rear gate will provide a more challenging extraction if the trailer is on its left side.
  - ▪ If a trailer is upright, offload through the rear door, onto a ramp or straight across into another trailer. This is the only time reloading onto another cattle pot is recommended.
- ○ Exercise full caution to be sure livestock and humans are not injured when opening the trailer. This includes the following:
  - ▪ Not cutting into or through livestock beneath where you are cutting
  - ▪ Cutting in a fashion so livestock do not have to exit the trailer on metal. Making vertical cuts so metal can be bent to the right or left, rather than horizontal cuts so the metal is bent up or down, typically is best. Wet metal or aluminum is very slick and dangerous. Make every effort to not have livestock exit the trailer by walking on metal
  - ▪ A multipurpose reciprocating saw (Sawzall) (Sawzall is actually a trademarked name registered to the Milwaukee Electric Tool Company [Brookfield, WI, USA] for this type of saw) typically is the preferred tool for cutting into the trailer. Using a lubricant such as vegetable oil will help the cutting process
- ○ Livestock generally will offload themselves if given the chance to settle down.
- ○ Offload as many livestock as possible before entering the trailer. If the trailer is on its side, it is useful to remember that the gates and ramps do not work in the same fashion as when the trailer is on its wheels.
- ○ Use humane euthanasia within the trailer only when mobile animals all have been offloaded. The use of personal protection equipment is paramount is this situation.
- ○ Humanely euthanize offloaded livestock that meet guidelines for euthanasia. Seek advice from a veterinarian or identified livestock person who has been trained in determining if an animal meets euthanasia criteria (broken limb, broken back, severely burned, badly injured).

## Relocation
- Preplanning is paramount to the successful resolution of an animal relocation. The authors highly recommend that relationships be developed before needing a location.
- Relocated animals need to be isolated/quarantined, especially those from an international origin or a sealed trailer.

- Biosecurity principles decrease the potential for spreading diseases. This basic methodology is founded on 3 tenants:
  - Isolate these animals from any other animal, preferably with physical distance separating these animals.
  - Prevent cross-contamination (feed and water) between the existing herd and these animals.
  - Limit unnecessary human interactions with these animals.
- Feeding management for these animals needs to be basic. Only provide good-quality hay and plenty of fresh, clean water. Avoid using grain-based feeds because the situation could be worsened by causing digestive disturbances.
- The health regimen and follow-up care of these animals need to be turned over to a veterinarian as soon as possible. Internal injuries may have a delayed presentation. Animals from the accident may need serial rechecks spanning from days to weeks following the incident.

## Transportation of livestock from an accident scene to a relocation facility

- Livestock should be transported to the relocation facility using a pickup and a stock trailer, not a semitrailer. Often in these situations, the size of a semitrailer makes it challenging to reload at the scene. As well, in the vast majority of cases a portable loading chute will be needed to reload cattle into a semitrailer. Finally, cattle with leg injuries will have difficulty walking up the loading chute and will have a more challenging time standing in the semitrailer. Most animals that have been extracted from a semitrailer will be resistant to reload into a semitrailer at the scene.
- Identify possible individuals who can transport livestock in advance of a potential accident. Detail those who can provide transportation on the "Call List." The dispatcher should begin locating individuals on the call list after an accident call comes in.
- Keep loads consistent until transportable animals are gone (avoid creating situations in which animals are left alone in the holding pen or on the trailer).
- Load density should be configured via industry standards and adjusted to meet unique individual accident circumstances (for example, animals with broken legs) (see **Fig. 4**; **Fig. 6**).
- Do not try to load livestock into trailers on pavement or concrete. If this is the only option, cover the roadway with sand or soil or a nonslip trailer mat at the entrance to the trailer. Livestock slip on paved/concrete road surfaces. When livestock slip, they (1) become scared, more agitated, and more dangerous to humans and (2) often become injured or more severely injured.
- If livestock need to cross the lines on a highway, cover the lines with sand or soil. Livestock typically will balk and not cross lines on a highway.
- Drivers should drive carefully, fully realizing that they are hauling scared and likely injured livestock. Driving precautions should include driving at a reasonable speed, taking corners easily, and stopping gently.

## Mortality disposal

- Plan ahead for dealing with mortalities and carcasses. Review the guidance on mortality disposal in Jan K. Shearer and colleagues' article, "Humane Euthanasia and Carcass Disposal," in this issue.
- Options for mortality disposal should be detailed in the "Emergency Contact Sheet" (see Appendix 1). These contacts should be notified early in the response process.
- The final disposition of mortalities needs to occur as soon as possible.

Maximum[a] number of head for trailers of different lengths for *polled & dehorned cattle*

| Width "ft" | Length "ft" | Number of cattle on trailer under, lbs | | | | | | | | | | Max[b] |
|---|---|---|---|---|---|---|---|---|---|---|---|---|
| | | 400 | 500 | 600 | 700 | 800 | 900 | 1000 | 1200 | 1400 | 1600 | |
| 6 | 14 | 16 | 13 | 11 | 9 | 8 | 7 | 6 | 5 | 5 | 4 | <6500 |
| 6 | 16 | 18 | 15 | 12 | 11 | 9 | 8 | 7 | 6 | 5 | 5 | <7400 |
| 6 | 18 | 21 | 17 | 14 | 12 | 10 | 9 | 8 | 7 | 6 | 6 | <8400 |
| 6 | 20 | 23 | 18 | 15 | 13 | 12 | 10 | 9 | 8 | 7 | 6 | <9300 |
| 6 | 22 | 25 | 20 | 17 | 15 | 13 | 11 | 10 | 8 | 7 | 7 | <10200 |
| 6 | 24 | 28 | 22 | 18 | 16 | 14 | 12 | 11 | 9 | 8 | 7 | <11100 |
| 6 | 26 | 30 | 24 | 20 | 17 | 15 | 13 | 12 | 10 | 9 | 8 | <12000 |
| 6 | 28 | 32 | 26 | 22 | 18 | 16 | 14 | 13 | 11 | 9 | 9 | <13000 |
| 6 | 30 | 35 | 28 | 23 | 20 | 17 | 15 | 14 | 12 | 10 | 9 | <13900 |
| 6 | 32 | 37 | 30 | 25 | 21 | 18 | 16 | 15 | 12 | 11 | 10 | <14800 |
| 6 | 34 | 39 | 31 | 26 | 22 | 20 | 17 | 16 | 13 | 11 | 10 | <15700 |
| 7 | 20 | 27 | 22 | 18 | 15 | 13 | 12 | 1 | 9 | 8 | 7 | <10800 |
| 7 | 22 | 30 | 24 | 20 | 17 | 15 | 13 | 12 | 10 | 8 | 8 | <11900 |
| 7 | 24 | 32 | 26 | 22 | 18 | 16 | 14 | 13 | 11 | 9 | 9 | <13000 |
| 7 | 26 | 35 | 28 | 23 | 20 | 18 | 16 | 14 | 12 | 10 | 9 | <14000 |
| 7 | 28 | 38 | 30 | 25 | 22 | 19 | 17 | 15 | 13 | 11 | 10 | <15100 |
| 7 | 30 | 40 | 32 | 27 | 23 | 20 | 18 | 16 | 13 | 12 | 11 | <16200 |
| 7 | 32 | 43 | 34 | 29 | 25 | 22 | 19 | 17 | 14 | 12 | 11 | <17300 |
| 7 | 34 | 46 | 37 | 31 | 26 | 23 | 20 | 18 | 15 | 13 | 12 | <18400 |

**Fig. 6.** Maximum number of head of cattle for trailers of different lengths for cattle without horns. [a] The number of head loaded during hot conditions should be reduced. [b] The maximum weight of cattle for each trailer size. Do not exceed Gross Vehicle Weight Rating for the truck and stock trailer.

- Animal mortalities should be handled with the same dignity and respect as human mortalities.
- Using visual barriers is critical. If swine are involved in the accident, the barriers must be of significant strength to stop the animals and keep them from chewing on or through the barrier.
- Tarps, vehicles, physical distance, crowd control/exclusion, various locally available methods can be used to help extract animals.
- Maintain carcass integrity to every extent possible.
- Various equipment, including heavy tarps, straps, and baler, mine and conveyor belts, can be used to help extract animals.
- Contact various state and local agencies that have additional experience in mortality recovery and removal from trailers.

**"Righting" of vehicle** The righting of the vehicle should be completed by trained professional personnel. These professional entities should be detailed in the "Emergency Contact Sheet" (see Appendix 1). The righting of the vehicle, especially cattle pots, will require heavy equipment and specialized training. This is one step that must be worked out ahead of time.

The vehicle should not be "righted" with livestock, alive or dead, on it (unless using specially trained, heavy recovery experts). The body of the trailer often has been damaged and cannot take the pressure of having livestock on it when being righted, and it will be damaged further. This scenario of righting a trailer with mortalities or live animals on it could be a very dangerous situation for livestock and emergency workers.

## Response checklist

- Close the highway/road
- Dispatcher calls entities on "Emergency Contact List"
- Containment facilities providers
- Veterinarian
- Relocation vehicles
- Relocation facilities
- Wrecker/tow truck
- Mortality disposal vehicles
- Mortality disposal facilities
- Scene secured and a perimeter fence built
- Scene and animal situation assessed
- Action plans developed

Make every effort to assure the safety of humans and animals before and during extrication.

## Containment misspelled

- Euthanize candidates for euthanasia using techniques described in Jan K. Shearer and colleagues' article, "Humane Euthanasia and Carcass Disposal," in this issue.
- Relocate animals.
- Relocate mortalities.
- Right and relocate wrecked vehicle.
- Contact load owner.
- Contact insurance companies.
- Detail all animals encountered on the "Animal Transport Incident Assessment"

## RECOVERY
### Debriefing

In the aftermath of a serious incident, many involved may not recognize the stress they are experiencing as a result of what they have witnessed. Stress can manifest itself in many ways. Debriefing is a method that emergency responders use to help relieve the stresses they may or may not recognize. Debriefing, whether formal or informal, should be conducted after every emergency response event.

For more information on debriefing and emotional and mental stress, see Erin Wasson and Audry Wieman's article, "'I Can't Stop Thinking About It': Mental Health During Environmental Crisis and Mass Incident Disasters," in this issue.

### Recovery Checklist

- Debriefing
- Submit invoices to insurance company or companies for reimbursement

## REFERENCES

1. Duckworth B. Truck accidents linked to early morning hauling. The Western Producer; 2007. p. 75.
2. Ontario Farm Animal Council. Undated. Livestock transport emergency guide. Ontario Farm Animal Council Bulletin. Available at: www.ofac.org. Accessed September 21, 2010.

3. Boyles S, Fike G, Fisher J. Cattle handling and working facilities. The Ohio State University Extension Bulletin No. 906. 2000. Available at: http://ohioline.osu.edu/b906/. Accessed October 10, 2010.

## APPENDIX 1: EMERGENCY CONTACT SHEET

| NAME | CONTACT PERSON | PHONE NUMBER |
|---|---|---|
| State Veterinarian | | |
| Livestock Veterinarian | | |
| Local County Extension Agent (if trained in livestock) | | |
| Local Brand Inspector | | |
| Local Livestock Transporter | | |
| Local Cattle Producer | | |
| Local Horse Breeder | | |
| Local Pork Producer | | |
| Local Sheep Producer | | |
| Local Poultry Producer | | |
| Local Bison Producer | | |
| Livestock Holding Facilities | | |
| Portable Corrals/Panels | | |
| Person Trained in Euthanasia | | |
| Dead Stock Disposal Facility | | |
| Dead Stock Removal | | |
| Tow Truck | | |
| Other Resources | | |
| | | |
| | | |
| | | |
| | | |
| | | |
| | | |
| | | |
| | | |
| | | |

**APPENDIX 2: ANIMAL TRANSPORT INCIDENT ASSESSMENT**

Responding law enforcement _____  Department _____

Phone _____  Email _____

Location of incident _____

Date/time of incident _____

**Transportation Company** _____
- ❏ Contacted
- ❏ Phone number_____

**Insurance Company** _____
- ❏ Contacted
- ❏ Phone number_____

**Driver name** _____
- ❏ Functional
- ❏ Nonfunctional

**Vehicle type**
- ❏ Farm trailer (bumper hitch)
- ❏ Gooseneck trailer
- ❏ Pickup with stock racks
- ❏ Bobtail truck
- ❏ Semitrailer (straight load)
- ❏ Semitrailer (potbelly)

**Vehicle condition**
- ❏ Operable
- ❏ Nonoperable

**Vehicle accident result**
- ❏ Upright
- ❏ On its side  ❏ Left  ❏ Right

**Accident site**
- ❏ Urban
- ❏ Rural
- ❏ On road
- ❏ Shoulder
- ❏ Ditch
- ❏ Other _____

**Animal type**
- ❏ Cattle
- ❏ Horses
- ❏ Pigs
- ❏ Sheep
- ❏ Poultry
- ❏ Deer
- ❏ Bison
- ❏ Llama
- ❏ Ostrich/Emu
- ❏ Other _____

**Emergency Contact**_____

**Comments** _____

**Age group**
- ❏ Young
- ❏ Intermediate
- ❏ Mature

**Quantity**
- ❏ Known  ❏ Number_____
- ❏ Unknown  ❏ Estimate_____

**Classification**
- ❏ Slaughter
- ❏ Feeder
- ❏ Replacement
- ❏ Biosecurity concern (sealed trucks, etc.)

**Destination**
- ❏ Farm          ❏ Auction market
- ❏ Slaughter plant   ❏ Feedlot
- ❏ Other _____

**Scene Security Status**
- ❏ Contained
  - ❏ Number tied _____
  - ❏ Number loose _____
- ❏ Escaped _____

**Health Status**
- ❏ Uninjured _____
- ❏ Injured _____
- ❏ Dead _____
- ❏ Unknown _____

**Extrication**
- ❏ Yes  ❏ No

**Support required**
- ❏ Live animal transport/relocation
- ❏ Personnel
  - ❏ Veterinarian
  - ❏ Euthanasia specialist
  - ❏ County Extension agent
- ❏ Equipment
  - ❏ Fencing
  - ❏ Gates
  - ❏ Lighting
  - ❏ Tow truck

22

## APPENDIX 3: CLASSES OF CATTLE

Appendix 3 details classes of cattle first responders may encounter, and their associated behavioral characteristics. It is important to remember, many trailers can have mixed classes of cattle and other on the same load, ie, beef cows, beef calves, beef bulls, and horses.

Also, these animals have been subjected to additional stressors and could react differently than the following generalizations:

1. Veal calves
   a. Small intensively raised animals often totally lack any avoidance (fight or flight) response
   b. Generally baby bull calves, weighing between 80 and 120 pounds
   c. Usually need to be carried or moved with solid panels by pushing the "wall" toward them. Hot shot use PROHIBITED!
2. Bulls
   a. May be aggressive and should be considered potentially dangerous
   b. Tend to have larger humps on their necks, testicles between their rear legs, will usually have thicker hair on their foreheads
   c. Can weigh between 1000 and 3000 pounds
   d. May have special insurance needs in cases of needed euthanasia. If possible, ask driver about insurance requirements for euthanasia
   e. Beef and dairy
      i. Beef bulls should be considered DANGEROUS; extra precautions need to be taken. Do not put yourself in situations whereby the animal can get to you to hurt you with its head, feet, or other body parts
      ii. Dairy bulls should be considered EXTREMELY DANGEROUS. These animals will meet the general definition of a bull, but will be patterned in the following:
         1. Black and white patterns, red and white patterns, brownish and white patterns, or deer tan to blackish colored; most dairy breeds have a concave facial feature between their eyes
         2. DO NOT ENGAGE THESE ANIMALS!
3. Cows
   a. May be aggressive and should be considered potentially dangerous
   b. Come in a wide assortment of colors and physical characteristics
   c. Will have an udder between their rear legs, but lack other distinguishable features
   d. Beef cows:
      i. Come in an endless assortment of color and size. They will be large in size (800–2000+ pounds per cow)
   e. Dairy cows:
      i. Black and white patterns, red and white patterns, brownish and white patterns, or deer tan to blackish colored; most dairy breeds have a concave facial feature between their eyes
4. Feeder calves
   a. Young cattle between 6 months and 1 year of age
   b. Generally weigh between 400 and 900 pounds
   c. May be males (either intact with testicles between rear legs, or castrated with no testicles between rear legs) or females (small udder between hind legs)
   d. Not often aggressive
   e. Will likely be scared, skittish, and wild
5. Finished feedlot cattle (often called "fat cattle")

a. Generally between 1 and 2 years of age
b. Weigh between 1000 and 1600 pounds
c. May be castrated males (no testicles between rear legs) or females
d. Not often aggressive
e. Will likely be scared, skittish, and wild

# Preparation and Response for Flooding Events in Beef Cattle

Wesley Bissett Jr, DVM, PhD[a], Carla Huston, DVM, PhD[b],
Christine B. Navarre, DVM, MS[c],*

## KEYWORDS

- Floods • Cattle • Shelter-in-place

## KEY POINTS

- Floods are one of the most common and costly natural disasters in the US and the economic impact of such large weather events on agriculture is huge.
- Solid preparedness plans will make response and recovery more effective. Developing local, regional and state partnerships and planning for cattle evacuation or shelter in place are key components of flood preparedness.
- Immediate response efforts should focus on emergency medical and euthanasia needs, providing water, feed and shelter, and inspection of the environment.
- Veterinarians should familiarize themselves with common post-flood diseases in beef cattle.

## INTRODUCTION

Floods are one of the most common and costly natural disasters in the United States and were the leading cause of weather fatalities in humans in both 2015 and 2016.[1] Nine weather events costing more than $1 billion were recorded in the 5-year period between 2012 and 2016.[2] The economic impact of such large weather events on agriculture can be huge. Leading this list is the state of Louisiana, which suffered an estimated $367 million in total agricultural losses due to flooding from 2 major disaster events in 2016.[3] In 1 month alone, more than $4 million in livestock losses were reported due to reduced farm receipts and increased production costs. The economic impact of flooding in 2017, largely a result of an active hurricane season in the Gulf of Mexico, is projected to surpass all previous records. According to the Texas AgriLife Extension Service, Hurricane Harvey in 2017 caused an estimated $200 million in agricultural losses alone, with more than $93 million attributed to livestock losses, which

The authors have nothing to disclose.
[a] Texas A&M Veterinary Emergency Team, Large Animal Clinical Sciences, Texas A&M College of Veterinary Medicine and Biomedical Sciences, 660 Raymond Stotzer Pkwy, College Station, TX 77845, USA; [b] Department of Pathobiology and Population Medicine, Mississippi State University College of Veterinary Medicine, 240 Wise Center Drive, Mississippi State, MS 39762, USA; [c] School of Animal Sciences, Louisiana State University, 111 Dalrymple Building, 110 LSU Union Square, Baton Rouge, LA 70803, USA
* Corresponding author.
E-mail address: cnavarre@agcenter.lsu.edu

included the loss of cattle, calves, and industry infrastructure.[4] According to experts, the number of dead and destroyed livestock was likely in the tens of thousands.

Flooding is characterized in 3 ways:

- Cresting flooding
- Flash flooding
- Coastal flooding.

Cresting floods are typically high-flow or overflow river flooding, which often rise slowly, allowing several days' to weeks' warning. Melting snows, large volumes of seasonal rains, and torrential rains from tropical storm systems can cause rivers to crest beyond their banks. Flash floods are quick-rising floods following heavy rain falls, commonly occurring where rivers merge. Flash flooding often poses the greatest risk to humans and animals given their sudden and often turbulent nature. Coastal flooding occurs when the rising sea level inundates normally dry, low-lying areas with seawater, often following storm surges due to hurricanes and tsunami waves.

Floods are also characterized by floodwater flow velocity. The National Fire Protection Association characterizes swift water flooding as those in which water velocity is greater than 1 knot (1.5 mph) and surface water flooding as having flow rates less than 1 knot.[5] Flow rate is an important characterization, because swift water conditions require specially trained and certified first responders to provide interventive steps on behalf of stranded livestock. Swift water conditions, in the opinion of the authors, also introduce an additional mechanism for injury of stranded livestock. Increased velocities can overcome an animal's ability to maintain its footing while also increasing the severity of injury when submerged objects contact stranded livestock. Increased velocities also amplify the effects of water-borne sediments on dermis of submerged animals.

Regardless of the mechanism, flooding can result in the displacement, injury, disease, and death of livestock and other animals.[6] Beef cattle are especially susceptible to flood displacement given their primarily grazing management systems. Lack of access to food and water, submerged fence lines and equipment, and exposure to sharp objects, hazardous chemicals, and electrical currents all pose serious threats. Ingestion of hazardous materials can also lead to human food safety concerns.

## PREPAREDNESS

In large-scale flooding events, it is impossible to prevent all losses, but advanced planning is proven to keep losses to a minimum. Solid preparedness plans will make response and recovery more effective.

### Planning and Protecting Financial Investments

The historical flooding occurring in the 2015 to 2017 seasons has shown that areas that have never flooded before are now susceptible. Changing weather patterns and changes in land use characteristics appear to be increasing the risk of being impacted by floodwaters.

Developing written emergency plans provides one of the best mechanisms for livestock operations and veterinary practices to mitigate flood risk. A history of flooding will be the typical reason for including this as a risk. The authors strongly recommend that livestock producers and veterinarians consult the local Office of Emergency Management or Federal Emergency Management Agency (FEMA) floodplain maps to determine if they are at risk. The FEMA Flood Map Center provides easy access to this information.[7]

Flooding can have serious economic effects on an operation through facility and equipment damage, loss of cattle, and decrease in animal health and production.

Producers should consider purchase of insurance policies focused on protecting their financial and historic investments in their agriculture operations rather than depending solely on potential support from the federal government.[8] Flooding is often accompanied by high winds and may damage natural and manmade structures. A detailed inventory list and photographs of equipment (including make and model), supplies, hazardous chemicals, fertilizer, and fuel should be readily available before and after an event. A detailed and current livestock inventory should also be maintained. Veterinarians can assist their clients by encouraging policy maintenance and helping to develop good livestock record-keeping practices.

### Develop Local, Regional, and State Partnerships

Cooperation with neighboring cattlemen and other agricultural stakeholders during the planning and recovery phases is essential, especially in wide-scale flooding events. Different tasks, such as livestock hauling; feed, fuel, and generator acquisition and distribution; and animal evacuation, rescue, and treatment can be assigned to individuals or groups in advance. Primary and contingent holding areas for evacuated and/or rescued cattle as well as staging areas and equipment needed for feed and fuel distribution should be identified in advance. A county/parish "feed bank" can be set up on high ground, and groups can purchase and share access to portable pens, chutes, and other equipment, such as air boats and high-profile vehicles necessary to get rescue or help shelter in place. Many local jurisdictions also allow prioritized entry for livestock producers so that they may provide care for their livestock.

### Maximize Herd Health

Cattle that undergo evacuation either before or after a disaster will be stressed and are likely to be commingled with other cattle. Herd biosecurity may be breeched. Maintaining cattle in good body condition and keeping vaccination protocols up-to-date is imperative.

### Animal Identification and Record Keeping

Disaster ready animal identification and record keeping should be part of normal operations. Copies of records should be stored in a remote location or in cloud-based programs. Access to herd records, proof of ownership, and registration papers may be necessary. Original papers should be stored in a portable, fire and flood–proof box that can be taken during an evacuation.

Should cattle get evacuated and commingled, or escape and are later captured, it is essential to be able to identify the herd of origin. Many cattle look alike, and plain numbered dangle tags and tattoos could be duplicated by other producers. Tags can also be cut out by rustlers, who may take advantage of disaster situations. Hot or freeze branding with a registered brand is the most foolproof way of identifying herd of origin. If cattle are not branded, producers should at least identify the farm or ranch on the dangle tag or use official United States Department of Agriculture (USDA) brite tags or electronic identification that is unique to each individual animal. Pictures and videos can also help with identification. In emergency situations where there is no time to uniquely identify animals, then the ranch name, location, and contact number can be spray painted on animals.

### Plans for Cattle Evacuation and/or Shelter in Place

Emergency plans for livestock operations that are at risk for flooding should address evacuation and sheltering-in-place. Some general considerations, regardless of decisions made about animals, are the following:

- Have a preselected site on high ground to move tractors and equipment out of flood-prone areas and away from potentially unstable structures.
- Store chemicals in a secure spot least likely to have water or wind damage.

Depending on the season, cattle may not be easily accessible if they have been moved for calving or grazing purposes. Although cattle will naturally move to higher ground when waters rise, they may not move to an area with an accessible escape route or that makes rescue practical.

### Evacuation

Beef cattle pose special problems when it comes to mass evacuation, so plans should be made weeks in advance of a potential disaster. Cattle evacuation may be possible either before or after an event. Decisions about which animals are a priority, such as genetically valuable stock or cows with young calves, should be made in advance for situations wherein it is not possible to evacuate all animals. Evacuation is much easier to implement when there is advance notice of an event and animals have been grouped according to evacuation priority. Prioritized evacuation may be difficult once rescue operations are underway.

Evacuation plans should include loading, trucking, evacuation routes (including contingency routes), and final destination. Well-designed penning and loading facilities will facilitate movement of livestock in as low stress an environment as possible. Portable facilities can also be preplaced or staged, allowing cattle to become familiar with the equipment before evacuation is necessary.

Potential evacuation routes should be developed with local, state, and federal road, bridge, and highway weight regulations in mind. The timing of evacuation is just as important as routes and destinations. Evacuation of cattle may not be allowed once mandatory human evacuation is declared. This prohibition may be instituted because of the potential for disrupting evacuation traffic flow, difficulties in obtaining law enforcement assistance with interrupting traffic to allow passage of cattle across roadways, and concerns over safety issues that may be encountered by personnel performing the evacuation. Travel speeds and therefore wind flow may be drastically reduced if evacuation of the general population is underway so transporting cattle should be concluded before human evacuation to decrease the potential for prolonged transportation delays, especially in very hot or inclement weather. The transportation conveyances to be used should be inspected before use and if possible be loaded in a manner to reduce overheating of transported cattle.

Identification of evacuation destinations should also be developed well in advance of flooding conditions. Prior identification of evacuation destinations is particularly important because livestock holding capacity provided by local jurisdictions may be very limited. Potential solutions to limitations in publicly provided space include identification of owned or leased property that is not in areas anticipated to be flooded and development of a list of potential evacuation locations that may be provided by the livestock community. Collaborating with other ranches to provide evacuation space will allow reservation of public livestock holding areas as a space to be used for rescued animals. Local Extension Service personnel can assist in identifying collaborating ranchers and livestock facilities. Veterinarians can provide a list of evacuation sites on their Web sites, in their offices, or in their practice vehicles for timely distribution.

Evacuating to other locations introduces biosecurity risks for both the evacuating rancher and the rancher providing pasture for emergency shelter. Biosecurity risks should be discussed as arrangements are developed and specific preventive steps identified and implemented before the comingling of livestock. Preventive steps may include disease testing requirements, vaccination strategies, or mechanisms for preventing comingling at the receiving facility. In situations such as hurricanes, where advanced warning is given, a Certificate of Veterinary Inspection (CVI or "Health Papers") should be obtained if cattle are to be evacuated across state lines. A listing of current state import requirements for livestock can be found at www. InterstateLivestock.com.[7] States may waive requirements for health papers in emergency situations. However, some testing requirements may be necessary before cattle reenter a state, and it is recommended that the state of destination be consulted directly when questions arise. Electronic record systems that allow sharing of information between cattle producers and veterinarians can facilitate writing CVIs in a timely manner.

Low-stress cattle handling is also a critical component of disaster planning for beef cattle operations. Cattle behavior can also drastically change following a flood or other major weather event, making them reluctant to be driven or corralled. Herds that are trained in low-stress handling techniques make rescue and movements before, during, or after an event safer and less stressful for both cattle and handlers. Being able to quietly move cattle may be the difference between life and death.[8]

*Shelter-in-place*
Shelter-in-place plans are often necessary as a result of the difficulties in transporting and identifying evacuation destinations for large numbers of cattle. Relying on shelter-in-place plans does result in an assumption of increased risk for loss of livestock.

If evacuation of cattle is not possible, they should be left in large open pastures. Confinement in barns and small pens or paddocks should be avoided because these conditions often eliminate the potential for livestock to move to survivable areas. Topography and flood maps should be used to locate the highest ground and cattle movement or transport to those areas planned in advance. A map of fences, gates, and roads makes moving cattle safer once floodwaters are present.

Effective farm and ranch maintenance plans will facilitate successful shelter-in-place operations. Minimizing the presence of equipment, supplies, and debris that may become airborne with high winds or encountered in floodwaters will lessen the risk for livestock, first responders, and ranch personnel tasked with providing care during flooding conditions.[9]

- Keep trees trimmed around barns, roads, and fences
- Keep tin on barns and shops secure
- Attach extra guide wires to augers on grain bins
- Maintain cattle trailers in good working condition
- Maintain penning and loading facilities in good working order and make fencing repairs in a timely manner

Providing fresh water, food, and shelter will be most critical immediately after a flooding event. Strategically locating equipment and supplies that cannot be evacuated to high ground will make shelter-in-place a more viable option. Items to consider moving to high ground include the following:

- Tractors and equipment for moving hay, repairing fences, and transporting livestock
- Round bales of high-quality hay
- Emergency water supply (used chemical storage tanks should not be used for storing emergency supplies of water)
- Water and feed troughs (these should be filled with water or placed inside of a livestock trailer)

- Fence repair supplies or portable panels (placed inside of a trailer)
- Hand pumps or generators should be available in case of electrical outages

**Supply list**
- List of important phone numbers (Appendix 1)
- Cattle inventory list
- Important maps of local area, including topographic charts
- Emergency supply of hay/feed, water, portable feed, and water troughs
    - A 7- to 10-day supply of hay and water is recommended
    - Large plastic garbage cans, which can be used to store small amounts of fresh water, but larger stores may be necessary
    - Instructions and chemicals necessary to disinfect wells[10]
    - Lightweight plastic swimming pools, which make easily portable emergency water troughs
    - T posts and wire to prevent helicopter from blowing them away, if plans are to air drop water from helicopter
- Fencing materials and portable pens
- Materials for portable shade structures
- Tool box
    - Hammer and nails
    - Wire cutters
    - Pliers
    - Pocket knife
    - Screwdrivers
    - Duct tape
    - Electrical tape
    - Spray paint/paint sticks
- Sandbags and plastic tarps
- Ropes and halters
- Leather gloves and rubber boots
- Gas-powered generator
    - All potential users should be familiar with safe generator operation[11]
    - The generator should be run under a load for a couple of hours at least every 2 months
- Emergency supply of fuel
- Blow torch
- Towels, paper towels, trash bags
- Flashlight and batteries
- Cash for emergency purchases
    - ATMs and credit cards may not work
- Emergency veterinary medical and euthanasia supplies
- Human first aid kit

**Preparedness checklist**
- Make sure family and farm personnel are safe
- Move cattle to high ground
    - If time does not permit, open gates and/or cut fences to allow cattle to seek high ground themselves
- Check emergency supplies of feed and water
    - Fill emergency water tanks with fresh water
- Move equipment to high ground

- ○ Set up generator in place before storm
- ○ Fill up all tractors, vehicles, generators and storage containers with fuel
- Secure equipment, logs, fuel tanks, feed troughs, and bins, and such, that are prone to floating or being blown away
- Remove shade cloth from portable shade structures
- Seal well cap and top of well casing
- Turn off water and electricity

## Share the Plan

Veterinarians can facilitate communication and be an integral part of the disaster planning process. Make sure all family and farm personnel understand the ranch plans and have plans of their own for personal and family safety. Make sure everyone knows where water and electricity cutoffs are located. It is advisable to also share the emergency plan with nearby ranchers and other veterinarians in case the ranch owner is unavailable during or immediately after an event.

## RESPONSE
### Immediately

Following a flood, downed and damaged fences are likely and cattle may not be contained in a safe area. Cattle that are roaming free could be a hazard not only to themselves but also to first responders as well as to motorists or others in their vicinity. A risk assessment of the surrounding area in collaboration with animal control or other emergency management authorities will help determine whether the animals can be safely contained, or allowed to roam freely in a safe setting until they can be corralled.

### Emergency medical and euthanasia needs

A quick inspection of the animals is needed to triage medical needs of the cattle. Some needs may be critical, and some needs may be able to be delayed until more immediate needs for water, food, and shelter are provided. Please see Jan K. Shearer and colleagues' article, "Humane Euthanasia and Carcass Disposal," in this issue, for euthanasia methods. Displaced cattle may become stressed and difficult to contain, and a perimeter fence or portable corral containing feed and water may be used to lure cattle in to a more concentrated area so that they can be evaluated. Sedation or tranquilization of an individual animal should only be done if it is severely injured, is in a hazardous situation, or poses a direct threat to people.

### Water

Fresh water is the highest priority even though cattle may be surrounded by water because floodwaters will likely have elevated bacterial and viral loads and may also be contaminated with toxic chemicals. Healthy adult cattle have about a 2-day supply of water stored in their rumen but after that they need access to fresh water. It is always best to provide free-choice water to cattle, but may not be possible. Adult beef cattle require at least 10 to 25 gallons of water daily. This amount may double in hot weather.

### Minimum water requirements

- Adult, nonlactating beef cattle: 10 to 15 gallons/head/d
- Lactating cows and bulls: 20 to 25 gallons/head/d
- Young, growing cattle (less than 500 lbs): 5 to 10 gallons/head/d

Getting fresh water to stranded cattle can be challenging. For small groups of cattle, lightweight plastic swimming pools make easily portable emergency water troughs, and large plastic garbage cans can be used to get water to cattle. For larger groups, large troughs are needed and water may need to be dropped from bladders by helicopter. Troughs should be secured with T posts and wire so that the helicopter rotor wash does not blow them away.

### Calculating trough capacity

If trough capacity is not known, the following formula can be used.

$$\text{Circular trough capacity} = \frac{3.14 \times \text{radius}^2 \times \text{depth (in inches)}}{231} = \text{gallons}$$

$$\text{Rectangular trough capacity} = \frac{\text{length} \times \text{width} \times \text{height (in inches)}}{231} = \text{gallons}$$

$$\text{Gallons by inch of depth} = \frac{\text{total gallons}}{\text{depth in inches}} = \text{gallons/inch}$$

Rules of thumb that may be helpful in providing water needs:

- 1 gallon of water = 8.3 lbs
- 1 cubic foot of water = 7.48 gallons or 62.3 lbs
- 1 gallon or water = 231 cubic inches

Contamination of water supplies can be common following disasters, particularly following flooding of water wells.

### Water disinfection

- Contaminated with bacteria
  - For stored water
    - Add 2 gallons of unscented liquid household chlorine bleach (5.25%) per 100 gallons of water
  - For wells
    - To disinfect water wells
    - Mix 1 gallon of household bleach and 3 gallons clean water
    - Add to well
    - Open all faucets and let water run until chlorine is smelled
    - Let the system sit for 24 hours
- Contamination with toxins
  - Have tested before providing to cattle or other animals/people

Flooding of coastal areas due to a hurricane storm surge can contaminate water supplies with salt. Dehydration, digestive upsets, and death may occur if cattle have been drinking water with high salinity, with calves being most susceptible. Lactation, hot weather, and exertion increase water intake and make adult animals more susceptible to salt toxicity if salt contaminated water is the only thing available. Signs of salt toxicity can also be seen when cattle are allowed sudden free access to water following an extended period of water deprivation.

Water salinity can vary depending on how much rain fall has diluted the seawater from the storm surge. Extension agents, Natural Resources Conservation Service, Navy, or Coast Guard personnel, may be able to help measure salt content of the water.

*Total soluble salts content of water (ppm = parts per million)*

- Less than 3000 ppm = Safe for cattle
- 3000 to 5000 ppm = Satisfactory, but cattle may be reluctant to drink, and it may cause diarrhea
- 5000 to 10,000 ppm = Avoid in pregnant or lactating cattle, old and young cattle
- Greater than 10,000 ppm = Unsafe
- If cattle have been drinking straight seawater (35,000 ppm):
  - Supply water with the salt content cut in half each day over 3 days
    - Approximately 15,000 ppm, then 7000 ppm, then 3000 ppm
  - Two methods
    - Mix seawater with fresh water
    - Add salt or electrolyte packets to fresh water
      - 1/4 cup of salt per gallon of water = approximately 18,500 ppm
- If cattle have been drinking brackish water with lower salt content (15,000–20,000 ppm) or have been without water for an extended period of time:
  - Try to provide grass hay first
  - Supply limited amounts of fresh water over 2 to 3 days
    - Ideally, water intake should be limited to 0.5% of body weight at hourly intervals until hydration is normal
      - 1/2 gallon per 1000-lb cow.
    - Try to ensure that no cows are overdrinking or limiting others access to fresh water
      - "Boss" cows that overdrink are a problem but hard to control

Conversion factors:
- 1 ppm = 1 mg/kg = 1 mg/L
- 1% = 10,000 ppm

*Feed*

Flood conditions often adversely impact available forage, and in the case of saltwater intrusion, may make available grasses toxic.[12] Cattle can survive for several days without feed, but a nutritional support plan will need to be instituted. The nutritional support plan does not have to provide ideal nutritional support because cattle can survive for weeks to months on limited feed.

Hay or grass is the safest feed source for cattle that are stressed and may not have had access to food for an extended period of time.[13] Wet hay is safe as long as it is not molded or infested with fire ants. Hay should be fed at approximately 2% of body weight or about 20 lbs per head per day. Other types of supplements should be avoided initially unless they are the only option. They should be high in fiber/roughage. After cattle have been consuming hay for a few days, other types of supplements can be added. Please see J.W. Waggoner and K.C. Olson's article, "Feeding and Watering Beef Cattle During Disasters," in this issue for more information.

*Shade*

Flooding events are often accompanied by high winds that damage natural and man-made shade structures. If this occurs during hot weather, every effort should be made to provide temporary shade to avoid heat stress.

*Environment inspection*

Damage to chemical storage buildings and fences may allow cattle access to toxic chemicals or plants. Cattle may consume plastic and metal debris, leading to digestive diseases. Fire ants and snakes are also common hazards encountered after floods.

### Immediate Recovery Checklist

- Inventory animals
  - Determine emergency medical and euthanasia needs
  - Calculate feed, water, and shade needs (please see J.W. Waggoner and K.C. Olson's article, "Feeding and Watering Beef Cattle During Disasters," in this issue)
  - Notify neighbors, brand commission, sale barn personnel of missing animals
- Inspect property for hazards
  - Debris and downed fences
  - Inspect working facilities before use
  - Identify chemical/pesticide spills or access to chemicals/pesticides[14]
- Inspect containment areas for fire ants and snakes

### Short Term

For information on carcass disposal, please see Jan K. Shearer and colleagues' article, "Humane Euthanasia and Carcass Disposal," in this issue.

### Decontamination

Decontamination is an important aspect of responding to flood incidents. Floodwaters typically have elevated bacterial and viral loads and may contain a variety of different toxic substances that may represent a threat to exposed livestock and the persons caring for them.[15,16] Contaminants may also pose a food safety threat. It is critically important to include hazardous material professionals in all aspects of decontamination planning and response because their subject matter expertise is necessary in keeping first responders safe, limiting the spread of contaminants in the environment, and guiding decontamination operations. A full discussion of livestock decontamination is beyond the scope of what can be provided in this text. The following discussion should be considered an overview.

Decontaminating livestock is a resource-intense event, and the decision to do so is best driven by knowing with certainty that an animal is indeed contaminated and the specific contaminants involved. There are, in addition, significant knowledge gaps and resource limitations that will make livestock decontamination on a large scale difficult.[17] It is ideal to know when decontamination efforts have completely removed all contaminants from affected livestock. Arriving at this level of certainty typically requires a laboratory diagnosis. There are typically not enough laboratory resources or financial resources to pay for them for this to be practical. In addition, laboratory diagnoses take time, and the decision to decontaminate or not is typically made in field settings and must be done in a timely manner. Floodwaters will likely be evaluated for bacterial and viral loads with pathogens of concern identified. It is completely reasonable to base decontamination decisions on water quality information provided by either public health departments or environmental protection agencies. If available, previous area assessments of nearby hazardous sites can be used to estimate the need for specific decontamination procedures.

Chemical contamination provides a more significant challenge in that a wide range of chemicals may be present in any flood situation. The types of chemicals that may be involved span the spectrum from household products to industrial chemicals. Although it is typically not practical to identify the specific chemicals that are involved, there are "tools" available to help guide the decision-making process. The first is US Environmental Protection Agency's Tri-Explorer Web site.[18] This Web site may be searched down to the county level and provides a list of toxic chemicals and their individual release amounts. This information may be segregated into facility-specific reports, thereby providing a reasonable list of potential toxic contaminants that may be encountered on a regional basis. The information that is publicly available is dated in that there is a 2-year lag time before the information is publicly available. Information of what may be released into the environment in a disaster setting should be incorporated into the planning process and hazardous material specialists consulted so as to develop plans that are likely to be effective and can be performed with minimal to no risk to first responders.

The second resource is the WebWiser program offered by the National Institutes of Health.[19] This Web site may be searched a variety of different ways, including inputting specific chemical names. The output provided includes information on the environmental fate of the chemical, safety and personal protective measures, recommended decontamination approaches, symptoms of exposure, and medical intervention strategies. Decontamination recommendations, symptoms, and interventive strategies are for humans, but the information may be extrapolated to the species that are impacted. The Web site also provides the ability to enter chemical characteristics, such as odor and appearance, clinical symptoms, or a combination of the 2. The output from this type of search is typically a list of potential chemicals. This list can be combined with local knowledge and information gleaned from the TriExplorer Web site to develop a list of the most likely contaminants and determine the most appropriate decontamination approach and the personal protective approaches required.

Protection of persons performing decontamination of livestock may range from simply paying attention to wind direction and distance from the contaminated animal to the use of highly specialized equipment developed specifically for working in hazardous material environments. A discussion of this specialized equipment is beyond the scope of this article; however, basic protective mechanisms are presented here. Basic protective measures to consider include the following:

- Eye protection: Safety glasses worn in combination with a full-face shield will prevent contact between contaminated materials and exposed skin.
- Respiratory protection: There are a variety of products that have been developed for protecting the respiratory system. They range from N-95 masks to supplied air systems. These products all require fit testing and participation in a respiratory protection program and are beyond what is typically available to veterinarians and producers. Use of a facemask will protect from inhalation of particulate matter and is recommended as a basic protective mechanism.
- Protective clothing and footwear: Protective clothing and footwear should preclude contact between skin and contaminated waters. As with respiratory protective measures, there are a range of specialized products available that have been designed for specific classes of chemicals.

Nontrained personnel should not participate in decontamination operations requiring more than the basic measures described above. In such cases, hazardous material technicians should be consulted before attempting any further livestock decontamination.

There are basically 2 types of decontamination approaches used. The first is a dry decontamination that is designed to remove particulate matter that reacts with water. Dry decontamination is performed by brushing or using vacuum-assisted equipment to remove particles from an animal's coat. It is not practical for range livestock but may be beneficial in cases of genetically valuable animals.

The second type of decontamination is wet decontamination. In most species it involves the manual application of soap and water to remove the contaminant. Many contaminants require multiple cycles of washing and rinsing to remove the contaminant. The most common soap used is Dawn soap, but other liquid low-concentration dish detergents can be used. Decontamination will also be difficult in range cattle and is likely to be reserved for genetically valuable animals.

### Flood-related injuries and diseases

Drowning, aspiration pneumonia, dehydration, submersion-induced cellulitis and dermatitis, lameness, and traumatic injury may occur when livestock are impacted by floodwaters. Sodium toxicity may also occur when floods involve brackish or salt water. The duration of time in which livestock are submerged in floodwaters will exacerbate clinical signs and prognosis. Floodwaters also may contain hazardous materials, resulting in poisoning through ingestion or contact. Ingestion of hazardous materials can also lead to human food safety concerns. The loss or inaccessibility of facilities and equipment can also inhibit or delay animal recovery and care.

The type and severity of flood-related injuries will be dependent on the ambient temperature and environmental conditions encountered during and after the event. Prolonged exposure to cold flood waters can result in hypothermia and subsequent decrease in metabolic and physiologic functions in cattle. The effects of cold stress can be exacerbated by wind and ambient temperature because wet coats will have decreased insulation properties, so cattle should be kept out of the wind as much as possible. Prolonged submersion in floodwaters commonly results in cellulitis and dermatitis. This condition is well described in the horse[20] and also occurs in cattle in the authors' experiences. The condition is characterized by a clear line of demarcation between submerged and nonsubmerged skin. Cellulitis and dermatitis are often severe to the point of intermittent to complete sloughing of affected areas. The condition appears to be quite painful and requires a significant amount of aftercare if a successful outcome is desired. Interventive care is characterized by initial decontamination, repeated cleaning and debridement, coverage with broad-spectrum antimicrobial therapy, pain management, and application of topical antimicrobials. Treatment is much more difficult in range cattle than in horses, particularly in disaster settings where there may be less opportunity to intervene than is the case in the equine population. A key factor has been the scarcity of livestock sheltering locations with acceptable livestock containment and treatment facilities.

Flood conditions also predispose livestock to infectious diseases. Beef cattle should be observed closely for signs of stress, injury, or disease for an extended period of time after a flood event. Although surveillance systems for most infectious livestock diseases do not exist, case reports of increased infectious diseases following floods or in flood-prone areas are well documented worldwide.[21–24] Anthrax may be a concern in endemic areas, because soil disruption and spore dissemination will be increased following flooding.[25] Similarly, beef cattle are at an increased risk for clostridial diseases, such as malignant edema (*Clostridium septicum*), red water (*Clostridium haemolyticum*), and blackleg (*Clostridium chauvoei*), because spores become more accessible to grazing cattle following flooding and heavy rain fall. Open cuts, wounds, and devitalized tissues resulting from flood injuries may increase the risk for spore entry into the animal. Cattle that die suddenly following flooding should be examined thoroughly and have a necropsy performed if the cause of death is not apparent or if disease is suspected.

Leptospirosis infections may be seen following prolonged exposure to water through ingestion as well as contact with mucous membrane or open cuts and wounds. In addition to acute clinical signs of leptospirosis, such as fever, anemia, jaundice, and sometimes death, cattle exposed to floods should be monitored for reproductive losses, such as abortions and stillbirths. Signs of aspiration pneumonia can occur 1 to 3 days following movement through high or turbulent water, and infectious respiratory diseases can also be seen at increased frequency when animals are stressed and commingled.

Both external and internal parasite control should be emphasized for an extended period of time after flooding. Population displacement and alterations in vector habitat may result in an increase in ticks and other insects. Biting insect populations, such as horn flies and horse flies, may also flourish and warrant targeted external parasite control.

Moist pasture conditions will also favor the survival of internal parasite eggs in the environment. Liver flukes, mainly *Fasciola hepatica*, are considered endemic in US coastal regions and the western states. Conditions favoring the development of the fluke, such as increased surface water and presence of the intermediate host snail, are found following a flood.[26] Intermediate stages of the fluke, which have burrowed into the soil, may also be disputed by flooding and increase pasture infectivity, resulting in increased exposure to grazing cattle. Acute disease from liver flukes can occur in a period as short as 2 to 4 weeks following ingestion of large numbers of the infective metacercariae over a short period of time. Moderate or continued ingestion of the metacercariae can result in chronic fascioliasis. Furthermore, hepatic lesions due to fluke infestation may predispose cattle to infectious necrotic hepatitis (*Clostridium novyi*) and bacillary hemoglobinuria (*C haemolyticum*).[27] An adult fluke can survive up to 2 years in an infected animal; therefore, continued monitoring and treatment with an appropriate flukicide should be extended for years after a flood.

Many diseases, such as leptospirosis, clostridiosis, and respiratory infections, can be prevented by routine vaccination of beef cattle. A comprehensive herd health plan should be discussed with clients in order to keep their animals protected before a disaster event occurs. If cattle were not previously vaccinated before a flood, timely vaccination of animals once they have been contained and given time to rest may be warranted.

Any lameness in cattle should be thoroughly investigated, because punctures, lacerations, and foreign objects can be easily acquired while cattle are moved through water with little to no visibility. Extended exposure to water tends to break down tissues and alter the skin's natural defenses, making cattle more susceptible to infections and physical trauma. Prolonged periods of time in wet, muddy pastures can predispose beef cattle to deep bacterial infections (deep pyoderma), cellulitis, and dermatitis as described previously, and infections of the feet and hooves such as foot rot, causing severe lameness.

Proper cleansing and lavage of wounds and punctures is necessary to prevent infection and more serious complications.[28] Lavage can be accomplished by using water or saline to reduce gross contamination, followed by the use of antiseptics, such as 10% povidone iodine or 2% chlorhexidine diacetate. Topical use of medicated ointments or creams may help clear minor dermal infections. Medicated footbaths, hydrotherapy, and systemic antibiotics are indicated in more severe cases. In all cases, care should be taken that any medicated products used are approved for food animal species, and that all withdrawal times are followed.

Mastitis can occur in beef cattle exposed to flood waters for prolonged periods of time. Cows should be checked daily, and calves should also be monitored to ensure that are able to nurse. Coliform mastitis, due to exposure to coliforms from contaminated waters, can cause acute septicemia and gangrene, and possibly death, if not treated quickly.

## SUMMARY

Flooding appears to be occurring at an increased frequency and severity, resulting in significant losses to the beef cattle industry. Responding to the needs of beef cattle is a resource-intense occurrence and beyond what can be provided by most local jurisdictions. It is incumbent on livestock producers to develop continuity of operations or emergency plans that are designed to limit the financial losses and compromised animal welfare that occur when livestock are exposed to flood conditions. Livestock producers and the veterinary medical profession should also encourage and participate in the development of public emergency plans focused on limiting losses in this critical industry.

## REFERENCES

1. National Weather Service. NWS weather fatality, injury and damage statistics. 2017. Available at: http://www.nws.noaa.gov/om/hazstats.shtml. Accessed October 11, 2017.
2. NOAA National Centers for Environmental Information. Billion dollar weather and climate disasters: table of events. 2017. Available at: https://www.ncdc.noaa.gov/billions/events/US/2007-2016. Accessed October 11, 2017.
3. Guidry K. Estimated impacts to Louisiana agriculture from persistent and excessive rainfall and associated flooding, August 2016. 2016.
4. Fannin B. Texas agricultural losses from Hurricane Harvey estimated at more than $200 million. AgriLife Today 2017. Available at: https://today.agrilife.org/2017/10/27/texas-agricultural-losses-hurricane-harvey-estimated-200-million/?_ga=2.140969142.544473965.1510868651-1684573131.1510868651. Accessed October 11, 2017.
5. NFPA. NFPA 1006 standard for technical rescue personnel professional qualifications, vol. 2017. Quincy (MA): NFPA; 2017.
6. Heath S. Animal management in disasters. In: Heath SE, editor. Flooding. St Louis (MO): Mosby; 1999. p. 57–67.
7. Interstate Animal Movement Requirements. United States Animal Health National Institute for Animal Agriculture. 2017. Available at: http://www.interstatelivestock.com/. Accessed March 7, 2018.
8. Gill R. Low stress cattle handling. In: Navarre C, editor. 2017.
9. Huston CL, Johnson KC. Hurricane preparedness and recovery for beef cattle operations, vol. P2507. Starkville (MS): Mississippi State University Extension Service. Available at: https://extension.msstate.edu/sites/default/files/publications/publications/p2507.pdf. Accessed December 10, 2017.
10. Gholson DM, Boellstorff DE, McFarland ML. What to do about coliform bacteria in well water. 2014. Available at: http://twon.tamu.edu/media/619641/what-to-do-about-coliform-in-well-water.pdf. Accessed December 2, 2017.
11. Thomas DL, Hannaman LM. Using generators for electrical power. 2006. Available at: http://www.lsuagcenter.com/portals/communications/publications/publications_catalog/disaster%20information/disaster%20information%20resources%20series/using-generators-for-electrical-power. Accessed December 1, 2017.
12. Twidwell E, Stevens JC. Dealing with saltwater intrusion in pastures and hayfields. 2006. Available at: http://texashelp.tamu.edu/wp-content/uploads/2016/02/procedures-for-feeding-rescued-cattle-horses-in-hurricane-affected-areas.pdf. Accessed December 2, 2017.

13. Anonymous. Procedures for feeding rescued cattle and horses in hurricane-affected areas. College Station (TX): Texas A& AgriLife Extension Service. Available at: https://texashelp.tamu.edu/browse/disaster-recovery-information/animals/.
14. Burns KPD. Pesticide storage concerns during and after a flood. 2016. Available at: http://www.lsuagcenter.com/profiles/aiverson/articles/page1473359201772. Accessed December 2, 2017.
15. Pardue JH, Moe WM, McInnis LJ, et al. Chemical and microbiological parameters in New Orleans floodwater following Hurricane Katrina. Environ Sci Technol 2005; 39(22):8591–9.
16. Colon J. Tests reveal extremely toxic floodwaters in Houston after Hurricane Harvey. 2017. Available at: http://wgntv.com/2017/09/12/tests-reveal-extremely-toxic-floodwater-in-houston-after-hurricane-harvey/. Accessed December 2, 2017.
17. National alliance of state animal and agricultural emergency programs emergency animal decontamination work group. Emergency animal decontamination best practices. 2014. Available at: http://www.cfsph.iastate.edu/Emergency-Response/bpwg/NASAAEP-Decon-whitepaper.pdf. Accessed December 2, 2017.
18. USEPA. Tri explorer. 2015. Available at: https://iaspub.epa.gov/triexplorer/tri_release.chemical. Accessed December 2, 2017.
19. Medicine UNLo. WebWISER. Available at: https://webwiser.nlm.nih.gov/getHomeData.do;jsessionid=EB082FB273399AB261C78C17161E3F58. Accessed December 2, 2017.
20. McConnico RS. Flood injury in horses. In: Sullivan EK, editor. Vet Clin North Am Equine Pract, vol. 23. Philadelphia: Elsevier Saunders; 2007. p. 1–17.
21. Wasinski B, Sroka J, Wojcik-Fatla A, et al. Occurrence of leptospirosis in domestic animals reared on exposed or non-exposed to flood areas of eastern Poland. Bull Vet Inst Pulawy 2012;56(4):51–7.
22. Ijaz M, Abbas SN, Farooqi SH, et al. Sero-epidemiology and hemato-biochemical study of bovine leptospirosis in flood affected zone of Pakistan. Acta Trop 2017; 177:51–7.
23. Parkinson R, Rajic A, Jenson C. Investigation of an anthrax outbreak in Alberta in 1999 using a geographic information system. Can Vet J 2003; 44(4):315–8.
24. Mongoh MN, Dyer NW, Stoltenow CL, et al. Risk factors associated with anthrax outbreak in animals in North Dakota, 2005: a retrospective case-control study. Public Health Rep 2008;123:352–9. Association of Schools & Programs of Public Health.
25. Griffin DW, Petrosky T, Morman SA, et al. A survey of the occurrence of Bacillus anthracis in North American soils over two long-range transects and within post-Katrina New Orleans. Appl Geochem 2009;24(8):1464–71.
26. Malone JB, Loyacano AF, Hugh-Jomes ME, et al. A three year study on seasonal transmission and control of Fasciola hepatica of cattle in Louisiana. Prev Vet Med 1984;3(2):131–41.
27. Kaplan R. Fasciola hepatica: a review of the economic impact in cattle and considerations for control. Vet Ther 2001;2(1):40–50.
28. Palmer S. Large animal first aid. In: Wingfield WE, Palmer SB, editors. Veterinary disaster response. Ames (IA): Wiley-Blackwell; 2009. p. 301–24.

## APPENDIX 1: LIST OF IMPORTANT PHONE NUMBERS

| |
|---|
| Emergency management |
| Fire and rescue |
| Highway patrol |
| Sheriff |
| Police |
| Animal control |
| Extension office |
| USDA Farm Service Agency (FSA) |
| USDA Natural Resources Conservation Service (NRCS) |
| Hospital |
| Utilities (electric) |
| Utilities (gas) |
| Utilities (water) |
| State animal response team |
| Extension veterinarian |
| Local veterinarians |
| College/school of veterinary medicine |
| Animal poison control |
| Local humane society |
| Cattlemen's association |
| Feed stores/suppliers |
| Fairgrounds/racetracks |
| Livestock haulers |
| Brand commission |
| State veterinarian |
| Volunteer list is attached |
| Resource list is attached |

# Managing Heat Stress Episodes in Confined Cattle

Kevin F. Sullivan, BVSc[a],*, Terry L. Mader, MS, PhD[b]

## KEYWORDS

- Heat stress • Cattle management • Environmental conditions • Animal welfare
- Shade

## KEY POINTS

- Cattle fed high-energy grain-based diets are at risk of succumbing to heat stress during heat waves incurring substantial economic loss.
- Deaths from heat stress are greater after several days of high temperatures, high humidity with low air movement, and only limited nighttime cooling.
- Respiratory rate, panting score, and behavioral changes are useful indicators of heat stress in feedlot cattle.
- Manipulating management of nutrition and feeding practices during heat stress events can reduce losses.
- Developing management plans for managing heat stress events proactively rather than relying on crisis management during an event is paramount.

## INTRODUCTION

Feedlot cattle consuming large amounts of feed and gaining rapidly generate significant amounts of metabolic heat. There are four ways cattle can dissipate heat from the body to the environment: (1) conduction, (2) convection, (3) radiation, and (4) evaporation (sweating and reparation).[1,2] The first three mechanisms require a temperature gradient from the animal to the environment; that is, the air around the animal is cooler than the temperature of the animal. At high ambient temperatures that approach or exceed the body temperature, the first three mechanisms are not effective, and the animal must rely on evaporative cooling.[3,4] However, if the relative humidity is also high, evaporative cooling is diminished.[3–5]

Diurnal ambient temperature patterns are also important. An animal can endure high ambient temperatures if heat gain during the daytime hours is balanced with heat loss during the nighttime hours. If nighttime ambient temperatures remain high, especially if

---

The authors have nothing to disclose.
[a] Bell Veterinary Services, 49–53 Dennis Street, Queensland 4408, Australia; [b] Mader Consulting LLC, 9301 Valaretta Drive, Gretna, NE 68028, USA
* Corresponding author.
E-mail address: DrKev.bellvet@bigpond.com

Vet Clin Food Anim 34 (2018) 325–339
https://doi.org/10.1016/j.cvfa.2018.05.001
0749-0720/18/     **vetfood.theclinics.com**

the relative humidity is also high, there is no time for recovery. In fact, nighttime temperature may be more important than daytime temperature in determining health and production.[4]

The impact of acute heat stress on livestock is well documented. Chronic, low-grade heat stress that occurs over several weeks to months in southern states is not well characterized. Chronic heat stress does not always show outward clinical signs but has the same potential as acute heat stress to impact the immune system and production. Climate change has the potential to extend impacts of chronic heat stress to more northern states.

## ECONOMIC IMPACT

Failure to dissipate heat in summer results in an accumulation of heat within the body and predisposes the animal to heat stress,[6,7] which may result in mortality, production loss, and substantial economic loss. Mader and colleagues[8] estimated losses from mortality and lost performance as a result of heat stress events to average between $4000 and $5000 for each animal that dies.

Since the turn of the century significant heat waves have been occurring almost annually in the Midwest and Plain states, with documented cattle losses up to 5000 head for each event.[1,9,10] In Australia, in 1991, a total of 2681 feedlot cattle reportedly died in a feedlot in Southern Queensland and in 2000, a total of 1255 feedlot cattle were lost in a southern New South Wales feedlot.[11,12] Overall economic losses from deaths and reduced performance from two events are estimated at US$28 million and US$40 million in Nebraska and Iowa, respectively.[2,13] In the summer of 2011, more than 10,000 head of cattle perished across five states as a result of heat stress.[14] The economic loss from reduced dry matter intake and decreased production is much higher than the direct financial loss from cattle mortality and is likely to exceed 5 to 10 times that of the death loss.[14]

Today there is an expectation that animals in confined animal feeding operations are provided not only food and water but a suitable place to live in comfort. Loss of healthy animals is unacceptable even in adverse conditions. Developing management plans for managing heat stress events proactively rather than relying on crisis management during an event is paramount.

### Factors Contributing to Heat Stress in Feedlot Cattle

Heat stress events causing mortality in feedlot cattle have certain environmental characteristics in common. Predominant are a combination of two or more of the following:

- High ongoing minimum and maximum ambient temperatures
- A recent rain event
- High and ongoing relative humidity
- Absence of cloud cover with a high solar radiation level
- Low, or the absence of, air movement over an extended period (4–5 days)
- Sudden change to adverse climatic conditions (lack of an adaptation period)

Feedlot deaths have been greatest after several days of high temperatures, high humidity with low air movement where there has been only limited nighttime cooling.[2] Feedlot mortality is highest in *Bos Taurus* breeds, cattle that are nearing finished weight, and higher performing cattle. Newly arrived cattle, sick cattle, and transported and handled animals (in ascending order of risk) are also predisposed.[2]

## Assessing Heat Stress in Feedlot Cattle

The ability to predict a heat stress event allows for preparation and mitigation of the effects on animal well-being and animal performance. An index combining temperature and humidity (THI) has been used for more than 40 years to assess heat stress in cattle. Although the THI is widely used in livestock industries, its origin is from research in dairy cows where it was developed to estimate the effects of hot and humid environments on milk production.[2]

Many THI charts have been developed for livestock and are used as a basis to provide warning or alerts signals for safe or hazardous conditions. An example of a THI chart is shown in **Fig. 1**. When the THI is 70 or less, lactating cows showed little discomfort. Feed intake and milk yield were depressed when the THI is greater the 75. Cows showed measurable discomfort at a THI of 78 and the discomfort became more severe as THI values further increased.

The THI, although useful, does not account for the effects of solar radiation and wind speed and does not include management factors, such as the effect of shade or animal factors (genotype differences). Solar radiation and wind speed may not be of much importance in a confinement barn, but are of importance in an open feedlot. To account for these factors a new heat load index (HLI) was developed by Gaughan and colleagues.[15]

HLI uses a combination of black globe temperature, relative humidity, and wind speed in the calculation.[16] The threshold HLI, above which cattle gain body heat, was developed for seven genotypes. Unshaded, black *Bos Taurus* steers have a threshold of 86, and unshaded 100% *Bos Indicus* steers have a threshold of 96.[17] Threshold adjustments were developed for various factors. These are shown in **Table 1**.[16] The threshold at which an animal gains heat is adjusted up or down based on these adjustment factors. Upward adjustment occurs when animals have access to shade (+3 to +7) and downward adjustment occurs when cattle are showing clinical signs of disease (−5). The positives are additive, but only up to a maximum of 96. Once an HLI of 96 is reached, *Bos Taurus* cattle gain heat.[16,17]

The amount of heat accumulated by cattle over time can also be calculated to acquire a heat load unit (AHLU) index. The AHLU records the number of hours over a day or days when the HLI is greater than the threshold value of the cattle. The AHLU gives a better indication of the level of heat stress than the spot measure of the HLI because it combines intensity and duration of exposure to the climatic conditions. It is then be used to calculate recovery time from a heat stress event. Once the HLI is less than 77, cattle can dissipate body heat to their surrounds.[15,17] Cattle that have been unable to dissipate all their heat through the night start the new day with carryover heat. These animals may be vulnerable to heat stress if the new day is hot. The calculation of the AHLU is based on measurement of the HLI over time in relation to the HLI threshold. An example is show in **Table 2**.[16,17]

Tympanic temperature (TT) has been used to study other factors contributing to heat stress, such as physical activity, season, and hide color. Physical activity induces elevated body temperatures. An experiment in which cattle were moved 600 m showed that (1) TT remained low and within a small range if there was no movement, (2) the peak in TT occurred 15 minutes after movement in the morning and 30 minutes in the afternoon, and (3) the time taken for a TT to return to normal was 3.5 hours after the peak TT in both the morning and afternoon (**Fig. 2**). When cattle were exposed to hot conditions in the summer, TT displayed a greater range than when cattle were exposed to cold conditions in the winter. Maximum TT was greater ($P<.01$) and minimum TT was lower ($P<.01$) in the summer than in the winter. Analysis of hourly data (**Fig. 3**) indicated that peak summer TT occurred around 1700, whereas peak winter

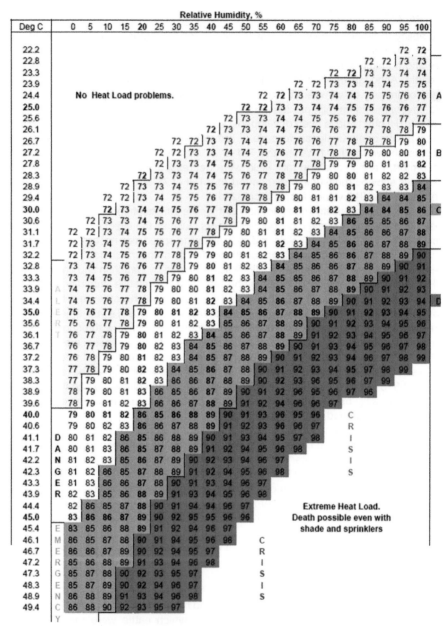

**Fig. 1.** Temperature humidity index chart. Alert phase- mild heat load effects especially on vulnerable cattle. Time to think about an implement heat load reduction strategies. Death not likely; Danger phase – strong to severe heat load effects on cattle. Death unlikely but possible. Sprinklers should be used judiciously at this time; Emergency phase – severe to extreme heat load effects on cattle. Death possible in vulnerable cattle without access to shade or sprinklers; Crisis phase – extreme heat load (EHL). Death possible even with shade and sprinklers. (*From* Sparke EJ, Young BA, Gaughan JB, et al. Heat load in feedlot cattle [report]. Meat and Livestock Australia Limited; 2001; with permission.)

**Table 1**
**The effect of various factors on the upper HLI threshold**

| Factor | Effect on Upper HLI Threshold | Factor | Effect on Upper HLI Threshold |
|---|---|---|---|
| *Bos taurus* genotypes | 0 | Manure management feedlot class = 1 | 0 |
| *Bos indicus* cross (25%) | +4 | Manure management feedlot class = 2 | −4 |
| Bos *indicus* cross (50%) | +7 | Manure management feedlot class = 3 | −8 |
| B *indicus* cross (75%) | +8 | Manure management feedlot class = 4 | −8 |
| B *indicus* genotypes | +10 | No shade | 0 |
| Wagyu | +4 | Shade (1.5 m²/SCU–2 m²/SCU) | +3 |
| European genotypes | +3 | Shade (2 m²/SCU–3 m²/SCU) | +5 |
| Black coat color | 0 | Shade (3 m²/SCU–5 m²/SCU) | +7 |
| Red coat color | +1 | Temperature of water in troughs = 15°C –20°C | +1 |
| White coat color | +3 | Temperature of water in troughs = 20°C –30°C | 0 |
| Days on feed (0–80) | +2 | Temperature of water in troughs = 30°C –35°C | −1 |
| Days on feed (80–130) | 0 | Temperature of water in troughs >35°C | −2 |
| Days on feed (130 +) | −3 | Install extra water troughs (emergency mitigation) | +1 |
| Healthy | 0 | Implement heat load feeding strategy (emergency) | +2 |
| Sick/recovering/ unacclimatized | −5 | Strategic clearing of high manure deposition areas | +2 |

*Abbreviation:* SCU, standard cattle unit.
*From* MLA. Tips and tools, heatload in feedlot cattle. Meat and Livestock Australia; 2006; with permission.

TT is not as evident. During hot environmental conditions, TT of dark or black-hided cattle is 0.5°C to 0.8°C greater than light or white-hided cattle from mid to late afternoon (**Fig. 4**). Cattle that are most susceptible to heat stress are therefore black-hided and cattle being full-fed a high-energy diet. Cattle nearly finished or carrying higher than average body condition are also subject to heat stress.

### Clinical Signs of Heat Stress

In people severe heat-related injury includes cardiac, renal, hepatic, and respiratory failure, and rhabdomyolysis, seizures, and diffuse intravascular coagulation (DIC).[18] In animals, clinical signs of severe heat stress are hyperthermia recumbency, tachypnea, open-mouth breathing, hypersalivation, tachycardia, dehydration, and a variety of neurologic signs.[18] Additional clinical findings include bilateral serous nasal discharge; increased bronchovesicular sounds; and cranioventral pulmonary consolidation, confirmed via transthoracic ultrasonography. Clinical pathology changes include markedly elevated muscle enzymes, increased blood urea nitrogen and creatinine, and hyperfibrinogenemia.[18]

Respiratory rate and panting score are useful indicators of heat stress in cattle because they are the first visual changes seen during hot conditions. Norris and colleagues[19] found that the respiratory rate of cattle increased by 5.7 breaths per minute for every 1°C ambient temperature greater than 25°C. Holt[20] used a simple panting

**Table 2**
**The change in AHLU over a 14-hour period, based on the reference animal**

| Time | HLI | HL Balance | AHLU |
|------|-----|------------|------|
| 8:00 | 85 | 0 | 0 |
| 9:00 | 86 | 0 | 0 |
| 10:00 | 88 | 2 | 2 |
| 11:00 | 92 | 6 | 8 |
| 12:00 | 94 | 8 | 16 |
| 13:00 | 95 | 9 | 25 |
| 14:00 | 97 | 11 | 36 |
| 15:00 | 96 | 10 | 46 |
| 16:00 | 89 | 3 | 49 |
| 17:00 | 85 | 0 | 49 |
| 18:00 | 79 | 0 | 49 |
| 19:00 | 70 | −7 | 42 |
| 20:00 | 64 | −13 | 29 |
| 21:00 | 62 | −15 | 14 |
| 22:00 | 61 | −16 | 0 |

*From* MLA. Tips and tools, heatload in feedlot cattle. Meat and Livestock Australia; 2006; with permission.

score to assist in the assessment of heat-stressed cattle. Gaughan[21] used a panting score system that was modified from Mader and colleagues[22] 2006. This scoring system is shown in **Table 3**. For each panting score there is an associated respiration rate.[20] Cattle with panting scores of 3.5 or greater are at extreme risk of dying if

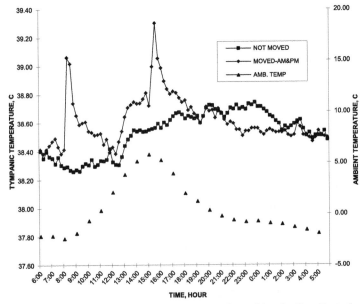

**Fig. 2.** Tympanic temperatures of cattle moved through working facility. (*Data from* Mader TL, Davis MS, Kreikemeier WM. Case study: tympanic temperature and behavior associated with moving feedlot cattle. Prof Anim Sci 2005;21:339–44.)

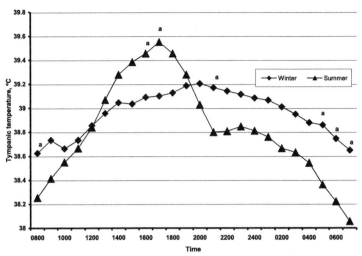

**Fig. 3.** Effects of season on tympanic temperature over a 24-hour period. [a] Means within an hour differ (P<.05; SE = 0.10). Each point represents the mean of 12 pens of cattle.[24]

they do not receive some relief from the hot conditions. The transition from a panting score of 2.5 to 4.5 can occur in 2 hours in extreme conditions.

Cattle progress through a series of behavioral changes as the exposure to excessively hot conditions increases to maintain acceptable levels of comfort. These behavioral changes are as follows[2,16]:

## Cattle Coping
1. Body alignment with solar radiation
2. Shade seeking
3. Increased time spent standing
4. Reduced dry matter intake
5. Crowding over water troughs

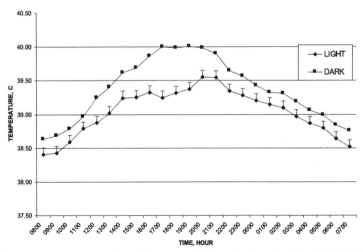

**Fig. 4.** Tympanic temperatures for dark versus light coat colored cattle. Vertical lines indicate SE. Means differ for 1200 through 2100 hours (P<.05).[24]

**Table 3**
**Panting score, breathing condition, and respiratory rate**

| Panting Score | Breathing Condition | Associated Respiration Rate (Breaths/Min) |
|---|---|---|
| 0.0 | No panting, normal<br>Difficult to see chest movement | <40 |
| 1.0 | Slight panting, mouth closed, no drool or foam<br>Easy to see chest movement | 40–70 |
| 2.0 | Fast panting, drool or foam present<br>Easy to see chest move<br>No open mouth panting | 70–120 |
| 2.5 | As for 2.0 but with occasional open mouth, tongue not extended | 70–120 |
| 3.0 | Open mouth + some drooling<br>Neck extended and head usually up | 120–160 |
| 3.5 | As for 3.0 but with tongue out slightly, occasionally fully extended for short periods + excessive drooling | 120–160 |
| 4.0 | Open mouth with tongue fully extended for prolonged periods + excessive drooling<br>Neck extended and up | >160 |
| 4.5 | As for 4.0 but head held down<br>Cattle breathe from flank<br>Drooling may cease | Variable ~ respiratory rate may decrease |

*Adapted from* Refs.[16,20,24]; with permission.

6. Body splashing
7. Agitation and restlessness
8. Reduced or stopped rumination
9. Bunching to seek shade from other cattle

**Cattle Failing to Cope**
10. Open-mouth and labored breathing
11. Excessive salivation
12. Ataxia/inability to move
13. Collapse, convulsions, coma
14. Physiologic failure and death

Cattle can usually cope up to symptom 9.[23,24] A sign that animals are failing to cope with the hot conditions occurs once cattle display behavioral symptom 10.

An early indicator of heat stress in fed cattle before clinical signs are noted is a dry matter feed intake decrease of more than 10% from the previous day, when cattle are monitored early in the morning. Additionally, if more than 10% of the cattle in the sentinel pens have a panting score of more than 2.5, heat stress should be suspected.

*Treatment*

In a crisis the opportunity to treat individual animals is limited. If the opportunity arises the use of ice cold enemas, electrolytes, and intravenous fluids using either normal saline or 5% dextrose and supportive therapy is indicated. Provision of cool drinking water is essential and together with shade and air movement is of considerable assistance when animals are exposed to high ambient air temperatures.

## Postmortem Findings

At necropsy, cattle that die from hyperthermia have sunken eyes and the body is hot to touch. Often there is bloody discharge from the anus and nares. Skeletal muscles are consistently glowing pink and dry rather than red-brown and moist.[19] Deep rectal temperature, deep muscle temperature, and body cavity temperatures are found to be consistently higher than 43°C. The heart is tightly contracted with epicardial ecchymoses and there is severe acute diffuse pulmonary congestion and edema causing the lungs and the mucosae of the trachea and bronchi to be dark red. Meningeal vascular congestion is seen when the brain was removed at necropsy. Cranial ventral pneumonia and fibrinous pneumonia are frequent although not always present on gross examination. Although not observed in cattle, Sula and colleagues[18] reported markedly enlarged and excessively moist pale kidneys in lambs that died from heat-related injury and the pale musculature that is seen in cattle.

Histologic lesions that are considered to be heat-related include acute renal tubular necrosis, pigment casts, tubular epithelial regeneration, multifocal myocyte degeneration, necrosis, and dropout with histiocytic influx and regeneration.[18] Bronchointerstitial pneumonia frequently seen is considered to be a predisposing condition to heat stress mortality. Rhabdomyolysis is a common heat-related injury in humans and domestic animals and is believed to be the direct effect of heat on monocytes.[25] Vascular compromise may add an ischemic element to the damage.[26]

## MANAGING A HEAT STRESS EVENT

When a heat stress event is occurring, the focus of the feedyard management team and the veterinarian must be on mitigation to prevent the situation from worsening and in managing the crisis. In most heat stress events there have been several days of adverse environmental conditions of high ambient temperatures, high overnight minimum temperatures, high humidity, and lack of wind speed following a rain event. During these days, the focus is on risk reduction and preparation for a possible crisis. The following presents a list of actions that should be considered to be implemented when a heat stress event is occurring.

### Cease All Cattle Movements

Physical activity induces elevated body temperatures. In summer, the rise in body temperature from handling can exceed 1°C for cattle with a mild disposition, but can exceed 2°C centre for cattle are easily excited,[27] so ceasing cattle movements is imperative. This includes all internal and external cattle movements, and all cattle handling procedures, such as processing, reimplanting, sorting, and revaccination. Pen riding, pen movements, and hospital cattle treatments should be ceased until the crisis has subsided.

### Water Availability and Supply

Water requirements increase with increasing temperature and increased water consumption is associated with increased evaporative cooling. So, water availability during time of heat stress risk is important. The relationship between ambient temperature and water requirements of beef cattle has been summarized by National Resource Council (NRC)[28] and is shown in **Table 4**. Watts and colleagues[29] estimated that in summer in South East Queensland water intake decreased from 14.1 L/100 kg for 300-kg animals to 9.9 L/100 kg for 750-kg animals. At environmental temperatures greater than 30°C, cattle tend to drink more often (at least every 2 hours) including at night.[2]

**Table 4**
**Water requirements of beef cattle in different thermal environments**

| Thermal Environment | Water Requirements |
|---|---|
| >35°C | 8–15 kg water per kg DMI |
| 25°C–35°C | 4–10 kg water per kg DMI |
| 15°C–25°C | 3 to 5 kg water per kg DMI<br>Young and lactating animals require 10%–50% more water |
| −5°C to 15°C | 2–4 kg water per kg DMI |
| <−5°C | 2–3 kg water per kg DMI<br>Increases of 50%–100% occur with a rise in ambient temperature following a period of very cold temperature (eg, a rise from −20°C to 0°C) |

*Abbreviation:* DMI, dry matter intake.
*Republished* with permission of National Academies Press, from Effect of Environment on Nutrient Requirements of Domestic Animals, Washington, DC, 1981; permission conveyed through Copyright Clearance Center, Inc.

To encourage water intake water troughs should be clean and recharged reliably. It is also important to ensure sufficient access. To meet the increased demand for water during heat episodes, Mader and colleagues[30] found that three times the normal waterer space (7.5 vs 2.5 cm of linear space per animal) may be needed to allow for sufficient room for all animals to have access. In addition to adequate space, waterers should supply at least 15 L/100 kg body weight of penned animals each day and should be able to meet the daily peak consumption needs in a 4-hour demand period. If cattle are bunched and crowding the water points, deploying extra water tubs (two or three per pen) decreases the crowding around the water trough and spreads them around the deployed water tubs. These tubs require continual monitoring and replenishing throughout the day and night. Supplementary water troughs should be filled predawn so the water is as cool as possible.

### Pen Surface Wetting and Sprinkling Systems

Feedlot ground surface temperatures can reach in excess of 65°C by 2:00 PM in the afternoon in Southern California.[31] Similar surface temperatures are found in most High Plains feedlots under dry conditions with high solar radiation levels. Cooling the surface would seem to provide a heat sink for cattle to dissipate body heat, thus allowing cattle to better adapt to environmental conditions. The benefits of sprinkling are enhanced if it is performed at night or at least in the morning, before the cattle get hot.[32,33] Elevated relative humidity may be problematic if large areas of the feedlot are sprinkled versus isolated areas in pens. Sprinkling small areas of a pen (1–2 m²/animal) does not appreciably raise humidity in a pen.[32] Intermittent sprinkling is recommended. Mader and Griffin[1] recommend a 2- to 5-minute application every 30 to 45 minutes or up to a 20-minute application every 1 to 1.5 hours. Other sprinkling regimes have been used including 5 to 10 minutes on and 15 to 20 minutes off, and a 3 minute on and 8 minute off sprinkling regime.[2] Mud build-up and up to a three-fold increased feedlot water usage is associated with a sprinkler regimen.[34]

Direct wetting or sprinkling of cattle can have adverse effects, particularly when the cattle get acclimated to being wet and failed or incomplete sprinkling occurs during subsequent hot days. It may also serve to further insulate cattle, diminishing evaporative cooling, especially on humid days.

## Nutrition and Feeding Management

Heat production increases with digestion and metabolism. This is known as heat increment. Heat increment are thought of as energy that must be dissipated. This is not really a problem under thermoneutral or cold environmental conditions. However, under high heat load, where the animal's ability to dissipate body heat is impaired, additional body heat may be detrimental to the animal's well-being. Feed ingredients differ in heat increment, largely because of differences in the efficiency of use of the nutrient or the end-products of digestion. For example, fibrous feedstuffs have greater heat increments (per unit of metabolizable energy [ME]) than feedstuffs containing more soluble carbohydrates. In theory, it is possible to formulate diets according to heat increment but evidence on whether this practice is effective in alleviating heat stress in feedlot cattle is inconclusive. The previous discussion suggests that in total the amount of heat generated from feeding a lower energy, moderate-fiber diet is more than that generated from a high concentrate diet. The addition of dietary fat seems to be the best alternative for reducing heat increment, because fats have a low heat increment. In beef cattle studies, mixed results have been found for steers exposed to high heat load and fed grain diets high in fat.[35] Neither has the addition of cations in the form of salts found to prevent or mitigate heat stress. Nevertheless, electrolyte demand is increased with sweating. With extended heat events, additional potassium and sodium may be needed.

## Pen Management

Proper feedlot pen layout and design are crucial for minimizing effects of adverse climates. Although cattle fed in areas that are not prone to mud do not see benefits of mounds inside feedlot pens, mounds have been found to be beneficial, especially in the Northern Plains and Western Corn belt of the United States by enhancing airflow during hot periods. If windbreaks are used, then wind barriers or other structures should not be placed near (~30 m from pen) cattle in the summer to maximize airflow in the pen and around the animal. Pen maintenance and cleaning are also essential to minimize dust or other problems that may exacerbate heat stress.

In wet, humid summer environments particular attention should be made to pen maintenance to ensure that the manure load in the pens is minimized. Pen maintenance should promote drainage in the pen and reduce the amount of water stored in the manure pad after a rain event allowing the pad to dry more quickly and reduce the potential impact of humidity in an adverse weather event. Pen cleaning should ensure that there is no more than 50 mm of dry compacted manure in the pen in the lead up to the wet season. A total of 50 mm of dry manure stores about 140 mm of water producing about 150 mm of wet manure.[24] It is recommended that manure depth should not exceed and average depth of 100 mm of dry compact manure during the dry period, remembering that a depth of 100 mm of dry compacted manure in the pen, 280 mm of water can be stored leading to 300 mm of wet manure.[16] The physical exertion of moving through muddy pens adds to the heat load risk.

## Shade

Shade has also been found to be beneficial for feedlot cattle exposed to hot climatic conditions.[36] In general, the response to shade is greatest at the onset of heat stress even though shade use increases as cattle get closer to finished weight. Shade improves performance in the summer particularly when cattle are fed in facilities that restrict airflow and for cattle that have not become, or had the opportunity to become, acclimated to hot conditions. Greater benefits of using shade are found in areas having greater temperature and/or solar radiation.[37] Generally, 2 m² or less of shade is not recommended and even though under extreme conditions welfare improved as the area of shade increased, 3.3 to 4.7 m² of shade per animal should be recommended for *Bos Taurus* cattle 100 to 180 days on feed because this amount of shade produced better welfare outcomes.[1,21]

## MANAGING A HEAT STRESS CRISIS WHEN MULTIPLE DEATHS ARE OCCURRING

In situations where deaths are occurring, the welfare of the animals is paramount and extreme mitigation measures beyond what has already been discussed may need to be put in place. These mitigation measures include

- Euthanasia
- Preparation of a mass burial site
- Postmortem studies
- Feed samples of the last ration fed and water samples
- Release of high-risk cattle from feedlot pens
- Early slaughter

Clinically affected animals should be triaged and those animals assessed as terminal must be euthanized humanely in accordance with the animal welfare policy of the feedlot. A method to dispose of large numbers of carcasses is necessary. This may take the form of burial, burning, composting, rendering, or a combination of these. Each of these methods of disposal has major logistical challenges and each method results in pollution of some kind. Burial may result in contamination of groundwater by the resulting liquid waste. Burning can create airborne pollutants and is visibly undesirable to the public and composting may result in surface soil contamination and potential runoff into watercourses. (See Jan K. Shearer and colleagues' article, "Humane Euthanasia and Carcass Disposal," in this issue.)

Postmortem studies should be conducted on a representative sample of animals. These are best done close to the disposal site. Findings should be recorded and pathologic samples of heart, lung, liver, kidney, brain, skeletal muscle, and possibly aqueous humor should be collected from a representative group of carcasses for diagnostic investigation.

Samples from the last ration fed should also be collected and retained for analysis at a later date if required. Water samples should be collected for analysis and water temperature and flow rate should be measured from several pens, especially those that have had high numbers of deaths.

It may be possible to release high-risk cattle from feedlot pens into the immediate proximity surrounding the feedlot if the ground surface temperature in the surrounding area is less than that in the pens, if additional shade is available supplied by trees or other physical structures, and if additional water is available and cooler than that supplied in the feedlot pen. Releasing cattle during the night or predawn when it is coolest and where the animals do not have to walk too far to the shade or relief structures is best. Consideration must be given to how easy or difficult it will be to retrieve the animals after the event has passed.

## PEOPLE

During a heat wave people are also susceptible to heat exhaustion, which if not identified and managed can progress to heat stroke, a medical emergency. If feedlot personnel are required to work in conditions likely to cause heat stress in cattle then strenuous work and light work should be alternated. It is essential that hydration is maintained. Wear suitable clothing and a hat and where possible work in the shade.

In a heat stress crisis that involves high levels of mortality it is important that managers are aware of the emotional and psychological capital used by caregivers working with the animals. Some people struggle to cope with high numbers of dead and dying animals. This also applies to personnel who are assigned the task of euthanizing animals during these events. It is important to provide access to counseling for personnel who have been involved in treatment, euthanasia, and mass burial of animals. (See Erin Wasson and Audry Wieman's article, ""I Can't Stop Thinking About It": Mental Health During Environmental Crisis and Mass Incident Disasters," in this issue.)

## SUMMARY

Heat stress is dependent not only on THI, but also on solar radiation and wind speed. Adjustments for solar radiation and wind speed have also been developed and need to be considered when predicting heat stress.[15,22] The effects of environmental stress are dependent on not only the magnitude and duration, but also on the rate at which environmental conditions change.

Losses of healthy cattle during adverse weather events should be small or nonexistent if adequate preparation and mitigation strategies are put in place. From an animal welfare standpoint, the use of shade or other mitigation strategies in the summer is recommended for most cattle that are confined and are on full feed, although in dry-cool environments in the summer, limited environmental stress mitigation is needed. However, with the current feed and cattle price structure, the economic benefits of minimizing the effects of environmental stress are greater today than in the past. In addition to the performance response, environmental stress mitigation has significant animal comfort and consumer perception implications.

## REFERENCES

1. Mader TL, Griffin D. Management of cattle exposed to adverse environmental conditions. Vet Clin North Am Food Anim Pract 2015;31:247–58.
2. Sparke EJ, Young BA, Gaughan JB, et al. Heat load in feedlot cattle [report]. NSW (Australia): Meat and Livestock Australia Limited; 2001.
3. Hahn GL. Environmental requirements of farm animals. In: Griffiths JF, editor. Handbook of agricultural meteorology. New York: Oxford University Press; 1994. p. 220–35.
4. Fuquay JW. Heat stress as it affects animal production. J Anim Sci 1981;52:164–74.
5. Mount LE. Adaptation to thermal environment: man and his productive animals. 1st edition. Baltimore (MD): University Park Press; 1979. p. 1–13.
6. Gaughan JB, Mader TL, Holt SM, et al. Assessing the heat tolerance of 17 beef cattle genotypes. Int J Biometeorol 2010;54:617–27.
7. Mader TL, Johnson LJ, Gaughan JB. A comprehensive index for assessing environmental stress in cattle. J Anim Sci 2010;88:2153–65.
8. Mader TL, Holt SM, Hahn GL, et al. Feeding strategies for managing heat load in feedlot cattle. J Anim Sci 2002;80:2373–82.
9. Hahn GL, Mader TL. Heat waves in relation to thermoregulation, feeding behaviour and mortality of feedlot cattle. Proc Fifth Intl Livest Envir Symp Am Soc Agric Eng. St Joseph (MI), May 29–31,1997. p. 563–71.

10. Hahn GL, Mader TL, Spiers DE, et al. Heat wave impacts on feedlot cattle: considerations for improved environmental management. In: Nienaber J, editor. Livestock Environment VI. Sixth International Livestock Environment Symposium, Louisville, Kentucky. May 21–23, 2001. p. 129–39.
11. Entwistle KE, Rose M, McKiernan W. Mortalities in feedlot cattle at prime city feedlot, Tabbita, NSW, February 2000. A report to the director general. NSW Agriculture; 2000.
12. Douglas I, Gibson J, Streeten T. Unusual losses in feedlot cattle at Texas, February 1991. Brisbane (Australia): Report, Veterinary Services Branch and Pathology Branch, QDPI; 1991.
13. Mader TL, Gaughan JM, Young BA. Feedlot diet roughage level of Hereford cattle exposed to excessive heat load. Lab Anim Sci Prof 1996;15:53–62.
14. Mader TL. Strategies to mitigate heat stress possible. Feedstuffs 2012;84:12.
15. Gaughan JB, Mader TL, Holt SM, et al. A new heat load index for feedlot cattle. J Anim Sci 2008;86:226–34.
16. MLA. Tips and tools, heatload in feedlot cattle. Meat and Livestock Australia; 2006. Available at: http://www.mla.com.au/NR/rdonlyres/4467D876-0499-4BA3-A940 943C1009E40D/0/TipsToolsRecognisingexcessiveheatloadinfeedlotcattlereprint Oct2006.pdf.
17. Byrne T, Lott S, Binns P, et al. Reducing the risk of heat load for the Australian feedlot industry. Final report. Meat and Livestock Australia; 2005.
18. Sula MJ, Winslow CM, Boileau MJ, et al. Heat related injury in lambs. J Vet Diagn Invest 2012;24(4):772–6.
19. Norris RT, Richards RB, Creeper JH, et al. Cattle deaths during sea transport from Australia. Aust Vet J 2003;81:156–61.
20. Holt SM. Feeding management to alleviate environmental stressors in feedlot cattle [PhD Thesis]. Gatton (Australia): School of Animal Studies, University of Queensland; 2001.
21. Gaughan JB. Assessment of varying allocation of shade area for feedlot cattle – part 2 (182 days on feed) final report. Meat and Livestock Australia Limited; 2008.
22. Mader TL, Davis MS, Brown-Brandl T. Environmental factors influencing heat stress in feedlot cattle. J Anim Sci 2006;2006(84):712–9.
23. Young BA. Implications of excessive heat load to the welfare of cattle in feedlots. In: Farrell DJ, editor. Recent advances in animal nutrition in Australia. Armidale (Australia): University of New England; 1993. p. 45.
24. Killip C, Smith L, Ceniork, et al. Managing summer heat workbook. 2014. Meat and Livestock Australia Limited; 2014.
25. Yarmolenko PS, Moon EJ, Landon C, et al. Thresholds for thermal damage to normal tissues in an update. Int J Hyperthermia 2011;27:320–43.
26. Olsen S, Solez K. Acute tubular necrosis and toxic renal injury. In: Tisher CG, Brenner BM, editors. Renal pathology with clinical functional correlation. 2nd edition. Philadelphia: JB Lippincott; 1994. p. 769–809.
27. Brown-Brandl TM. Heat stress in feedlot cattle. CAB reviews: perspectives in agriculture, veterinary science, nutrition and natural resources. vol. 3. Boston (MA): Cabi; 2008. p. 16.
28. NRC. Effect of environment of nutrient requirements of domestic animals. Washington, DC: National Academy Press; 1981.
29. Watts PJ, Tucker RW, Casey KD. Water system design. In: Proc Designing Better Feedlots Conference. Brisbane: Sunshine Coast, QDPI; September 22–23, 1993.

30. Mader TL, Fell LR, McPhee MJ. Behavior response of non-Brahman cattle to shade in commercial feedlots. Proc 5th Int Livest Symp Amer Soc Agri Eng. St Joseph (MI), May 29–31, 1997b. p. 795–802.
31. Kelly CF, Bond TE, Ittner NR. Thermal design of livestock shades. Agr Eng 1950; 30:601–6.
32. Davis MS, Mader TL, Holt SM, et al. Strategies to reduce feedlot cattle heat stress: effects on tympanic temperature. J Anim Sci 2003;81:649–61.
33. Holt SM, Gaughan JB, Mader TL, et al. Time of cooling important for cattle heat load alleviation. J Anim Sci 1998;76:97.
34. Gaughan JB, Mader TL, Holt SM. Cooling and feeding strategies to reduce heat load of grain fed beef cattle in intensive housing. Livest Sci 2008;113:226–33.
35. Gaughan JB, Mader TL. Effects of sodium chloride and fat supplementation on finishing steers exposed to hot and cold conditions. J Anim Sci 2009;87:612–21.
36. Mader TL, Dahlquist JM, Hahn GL, et al. Shade and wind barrier effects on summer time feedlot cattle performance. J Anim Sci 1999;77:2065–72.
37. Mitlöhner JL, Morrow JW, Dailey SC, et al. Shade and water misting effects on behavior, physiology, performance and carcass traits of heat-stressed feedlot cattle. J Anim Sci 2001;79:2327–35.

# Foreign Animal Disease Outbreaks

Danelle A. Bickett-Weddle, DVM, MPH, PhD[a],*, Michael W. Sanderson, DVM, MS[b],
Elizabeth J. Parker, DVM[c]

## KEYWORDS

- Foreign animal diseases • Veterinarians • Preparedness • Biosecurity
- Secure beef supply plan

## KEY POINTS

- Veterinarians play a vital role in recognizing and promptly reporting diseases or syndromes of concern in an effort to minimize the impact of foreign animal diseases (FADs).
- Private practice veterinarians are a tremendous resource for their clients and local community preparing for and responding to an FAD outbreak.
- Numerous resources exist for veterinarians to train themselves about foreign animal diseases, animal health emergencies, and help their clients prepare and develop biosecurity and business continuity plans.
- An FAD outbreak will require a concerted effort by producers, veterinarians, emergency responders, and state and federal officials to successfully control and eradicate the disease.
- Be part of the success; start preparing today.

## INTRODUCTION

A foreign animal disease (FAD) incursion affecting beef cattle in the United States is plausible due to global trade trends and increased movement of animals, people, pathogens, and feedstuffs. Areas of geopolitical conflict have also contributed to an increased movement of FADs out of their historical regions. Several important outbreaks have occurred globally in areas once considered free, including foot-and-mouth disease (FMD), lumpy skin disease, and HoBi-like virus.[1,2] An FAD is defined as "a terrestrial animal disease or pest, or an aquatic animal disease or pest, not known to exist in the U.S. or its territories."[3] The list of FADs (and domestically important diseases) affecting cattle can be found in the US National List of Reportable

The authors have nothing to disclose.
[a] Center for Food Security and Public Health, Iowa State University, Ames, IA, USA;
[b] Epidemiology & Beef Production, Center for Outcomes Research & Epidemiology, Kansas State University, Manhattan, KS, USA; [c] AgriLife Research, Texas A&M University, College Station, TX, USA
* Corresponding author.
E-mail address: dbw@iastate.edu

Vet Clin Food Anim 34 (2018) 341–354
https://doi.org/10.1016/j.cvfa.2018.02.005
0749-0720/18/© 2018 Elsevier Inc. All rights reserved.

*Animal Diseases*, available at: https://www.aphis.usda.gov/aphis/ourfocus/animal health/program-overview/ct_national_list_reportable_animal_diseases.

In response to the increase in FAD outbreaks worldwide, the US Department of Agriculture (USDA) Animal and Plant Health Inspection Service (APHIS) continues to develop and update the FAD Preparedness and Response Plan (PReP). This diverse portfolio includes strategic plans, emergency management guidelines, disease response plans, and the Secure Food Supply Plans for cattle, pigs, and poultry. The FAD PReP goals of an FAD response are to detect, control, and contain an incursion of an FAD in the United States as quickly as possible, then eradicate the disease using science-based and risk-based measures, as well as strategies that facilitate continuity of business for noninfected animals or noncontaminated animal products.[4] In addition to planning for a potential FAD incursion, the USDA has also developed guidance for emerging diseases, as described in the *Emerging Animal Disease Preparedness and Response Plan*, July 2017 available at: https://www.aphis.usda.gov/animal_health/ downloads/emerging-dis-framework-plan.pdf. These diseases could have a major impact on American livestock production, the livelihood of producers and veterinarians, animal and public health, food safety, food security, export markets, and the economy. Veterinarians play a vital role in recognizing and promptly reporting diseases or syndromes of concern in an effort to minimize the impact.

## ROLE OF THE VETERINARIAN IN FOREIGN ANIMAL DISEASE INVESTIGATIONS

Daily interactions with cattle across a community, state, or region allows veterinarians to see a variety of health challenges, recognize trends or seasonality issues, gather and share knowledge on successful treatment protocols, and educate producers about best practices. This broad exposure also puts veterinarians in a critical role: diagnostician for endemic and possible FADs. It is a tremendous responsibility and there are tools available to help refine clinical sign recognition for FADs and enhance preparedness for veterinarians and their clients. Many are described in this article.

"Early identification and quick response in the FAD investigations are critical steps to ensuring that any further spread is minimized."[5] Cattle veterinarians play a crucial role in this process. Whether prompted by a call from a client with concerns that the cattle seem "off" or blatant clinical signs that match the textbook and Web images from veterinary school, it is important to say something when you see something. Veterinarians should not submit laboratory samples or attempt to diagnose a suspected FAD on their own. It just takes a phone call. The steps in an FAD investigation include

- Call the state animal health official (SAHO) and the USDA assistant district director.
  - These individuals will discuss the veterinarian's observations and gather some history of the operation and the situation of concern.
  - If their suspicions include an FAD, they will then send an FAD diagnostician (FADD) to the operation to investigate further. FADDs are veterinarians employed by a state or the USDA who have had additional training in disease recognition, sample collection, and biosecurity to contain disease.
  - Depending on the disease of concern, the SAHO may recommend meeting the FADD at the operation or follow specific biosecurity measures, which may or may not include seeing additional animals that day (see later discussion on business continuity for veterinary practices).
  - A list of SAHOs is available on the US Animal Health Association Web site, available at: http://www.usaha.org/federal-and-state-animal-health.

- ○ A list of USDA assistant district directors is available at: http://www.aphis. usda.gov/aphis/ourfocus/animalhealth/nvap/NVAP-Reference-Guide/Appendix/ APHIS-VS-District-Offices.
- The FADD will arrive at the operation, interview the producer (and, possibly, the veterinarian), examine the herd, and collect antemortem and postmortem samples as needed.
  - ○ Between 2007 and 2016 there were over 5000 foreign animal or emerging disease investigations. Each year, there were 30 to 150 investigations in bovids, often with vesicular lesions.[6] There were several vesicular stomatitis (VS) incidents within that time span; however, VS cannot be distinguished clinically from foot and mouth disease (FMD) without testing. The suspect FAD call made by a veterinarian could lead to early identification, allowing control efforts to prevent spread and decrease the impact on animal health in that community and the country.
- The FADD advises the producer on appropriate biosecurity and containment measures to prevent disease spread while waiting for test results.
  - ○ The intensity of biosecurity measures will depend on the disease of concern.
  - ○ This may include ensuring only clean clothing and footwear leave the operation and making sure equipment and vehicles leaving are cleaned and disinfected.
  - ○ This may include issuing a quarantine for the premises when a highly suspect, contagious FAD is on the differential list, even before laboratory confirmation.
- Samples are submitted to the USDA National Veterinary Services Laboratories.
  - ○ Depending on the disease of concern, the samples are sent with varying levels of priority to a laboratory that is proficient in testing for that virus, bacterium, or prion.
  - ○ If a sample is negative for the disease of concern, the FAD investigation ends. Any quarantine or movement restrictions are lifted.
    - ■ The costs for FAD testing and investigation are paid for by the government.
    - ■ If additional diagnostics are needed to uncover the cause for the illness or death, those costs are the responsibility of the producer or the submitting veterinarian.
  - ○ If a sample is positive for the disease of concern, disease control and response efforts commence by the state and federal animal health authorities. The remainder of this article focuses on veterinarians and their clients preparing for and responding to an FAD outbreak.

When an FAD is confirmed, there are a series of events that occur:

- The USDA APHIS is the lead federal agency managing the outbreak, working closely with SAHOs, who have quarantine authority.
- The USDA notifies the World Organization for Animal Health (OIE) of the situation. More information on the OIE can be found at: www.oie.int
  - ○ The United States is an OIE member country and follows the guidance in the OIE Terrestrial Animal Health Code with respect to the safe trade of animals and their products internationally. The diseases in the Terrestrial Animal Health Code are included in the US National List of Reportable Animal Diseases with the goal of consistent reporting from US veterinarians and diagnostic laboratories.
- The USDA and the SAHOs work to contain, control, and eradicate the disease in an effort to protect animal health, public health, animal agriculture, the environment, the food supply, and the US economy (see later discussion).
  - ○ Operations with a positive FAD diagnosis will be placed under quarantine, imposed by the SAHO or, in a federally declared emergency, the US Secretary of Agriculture.

- Trading partner countries could initiate trade embargos for US animals and animal products due to international pathogen spread concerns. For example, if FMD is diagnosed, the beef industry will feel the immediate impact of lost trade of animals, meat, semen, embryos, and the numerous products made from cattle.

## ROLE OF FEDERAL AUTHORITIES, STATES, AND THE PRIVATE SECTOR IN A FOREIGN ANIMAL DISEASE OUTBREAK

The US emergency response to FAD emergencies involves a partnership between various government (federal, state, tribal, local) and private sector (industry, veterinarians) entities. An effective FMD response in particular will require collaborations on the broadest scale. The United States follows an incident command system (ICS) organizational structure and the National Incident Management System for FADs, which provides a common, nationwide approach to enable the whole community to more effectively work together to manage major threats and hazards.[7] The practicing veterinarian plays a vital role no matter the specific FAD or size of the event. If interested in the ICS, veterinarians can train to serve as group supervisors, team leaders, and team members to more proactively assist clients and community.[8]

The USDA APHIS is the lead federal agency for incident management during an FAD event involving livestock. As the incident grows in significance (eg, extent, risk), involvement of federal resources and entities increases. APHIS remains the overall lead when support is requested from other federal departments or agencies.[3]

- Numerous non-FAD outbreaks, such as tuberculosis or brucellosis, are routinely handled at the local level by the state animal health authorities, and cattle veterinarians often have an active role in the control and response efforts. The skills of practitioners will also be vital in an FAD outbreak. Livestock and mixed animal veterinarians are the daily boots on the ground whose local knowledge of livestock operations, livestock markets, and available resources could provide valuable insight to officials managing an outbreak, as well as speed up a response. In a large outbreak, state and federal human resources will be quickly overwhelmed. Some diseases, such as FMD, may take an extended period of time to control.

It is difficult to predict how quickly a US FMD outbreak could be eradicated. A Midwest FMD outbreak model showed variable results, with median outbreak duration from 181 to 527 days depending on the control scenario, and a range of 100 to 700 days.[9] Preliminary model data from a within-feedlot FMD model indicates the total time from initial FMD infection until the last calf is recovered in a large feedlot may extend for 60 to 100 days.[9] OIE guidelines indicate a minimum of 3 to 6 months of negative surveillance, depending on the control strategy, after the last case of disease before FMD-free status can be regained.[10] The time until the United States regains FMD-free status and until trading partners allow trade in beef products to resume will be longer.

Meanwhile, producers with cattle that have no evidence of infection will want to continue business operations. Private veterinarians will be a tremendous resource for those clients.

## PREPARING FOR AND RAPIDLY IDENTIFYING A FOREIGN ANIMAL DISEASE INCURSION
### Preparing Veterinarians

Veterinarians can prepare for an FAD in a variety of ways:

- As a diagnostician, stay current on clinical signs and syndromes suggestive of FADs (**Table 1**).

**Table 1**
**Training opportunities for veterinarians**

| FADs | Format | More Information |
|---|---|---|
| Center for Food Security and Public Health at Iowa State University Disease Image Database | Online, self-study | http://www.cfsph.iastate.edu/ DiseaseInfo/disease-images.php |
| Colorado State University FAD Training Course | In-person | http://csu-cvmbs.colostate.edu/Pages/ default.aspx |
| Emerging and Exotic Diseases of Animals Course | Online, self-study | http://www.cfsph.iastate.edu/EEDA-Course |
| European Commission for the Control of Foot-and-Mouth Disease FMD Courses, Lesion Library | Online, self-study | https://eufmdlearning.works/ |
| US National List of Reportable Animal Diseases | Online, self-study | https://www.aphis.usda.gov/aphis/ ourfocus/animalhealth/program-overview/ct_national_list_ reportable_animal_diseases |
| US Animal Health Association, Foreign Animal Diseases Textbook | Online, self-study | https://www.aphis.usda.gov/ emergency_response/downloads/ nahems/fad.pdf |
| USDA National Veterinary Accreditation Program (NVAP) Module 3: Foreign Animal, Program, and Reportable Diseases | Online, self-study | https://www.aphis.usda.gov/aphis/ ourfocus/animalhealth/nvap/CT_ aast |
| USDA NVAP Module 5: Vesicular Diseases | Online, self-study | https://www.aphis.usda.gov/aphis/ ourfocus/animalhealth/nvap/CT_ aast |
| **First Responder** | **Format** | **More Information** |
| USDA National Animal Health Emergency Response Corps Training Web site | Online, self-study | http://naherc.cfsph.iastate.edu/ |
| USDA NVAP Module 19: Animal Health Emergency Response | Online, self-study | https://www.aphis.usda.gov/aphis/ ourfocus/animalhealth/nvap/CT_ aast |
| USDA Training and Exercise Program (Series of Applicable Webinars) | Online, self-study | https://www.aphis.usda.gov/aphis/ ourfocus/animalhealth/training-and-development/ct_vs_training_ and_exercise_plan |

- As a first responder in an outbreak, take training courses about animal health emergencies (see **Table 1**).
- As a trusted advisor, help clients:
  - Prevent endemic and FAD disease introductions in their operations by developing ranch-specific or farm-specific biosecurity plans as part of daily overall herd health management, and encourage implementation as a routine part of prevention.
  - Initiate FAD business continuity planning by developing enhanced biosecurity, surveillance, and contingency plans.
- As practice owners or associates, plan for clinic business continuity by developing practice biosecurity and contingency plans.
- As a community member, get involved in local preparedness and response planning.

### Preparing Clients: Business Continuity Planning

Veterinarians can have a substantial role in helping their beef clients prepare for an FAD outbreak and maintaining continuity of business in the face of one. Specifically for FMD, before a US outbreak, veterinarians can assist their livestock clients to produce business continuity plans that are ready for implementation should FMD ever be introduced. Continuity of business during an FMD outbreak relies on the ability to move animals between production premises and to processing facilities. The USDA Secure Beef Supply (SBS) Plan provides a workable business continuity plan for beef premises, with no evidence of FMD infection, and for allied industries. Veterinarians play a critical role in the SBS Plan with respect to preparedness and response. The voluntary SBS Plan gives veterinarians the tools they need to help their clients implement key business continuity strategies.[11] More information about the SBS Plan is available at www.securebeef.org.

In an outbreak, the ability of beef producers to continue normal business practices will be based on where their cattle are in relation to infected herds and the preparedness steps they took before the outbreak. Although producers cannot control the location of the outbreak, they can take control of their preparedness. Producers have a responsibility to protect their animals from becoming infected, focusing on what they can control on their operation. Business continuity plans should:

- Include a national Premises Identification Number (PIN); producers request PINS from the office of their SAHO.
  - If producers do not already have a PIN, it should be requested from the office of their SAHO.
  - The PIN should be for the actual location of the cattle, not the client's home residence. Cattle producers with animals in more than one location are encouraged to have a PIN for each location that is epidemiologically distinct.
  - Herds with PINs established before an FAD event will significantly enhance the ability to rapidly track livestock origin and destination and potential infection.
- Minimize the risk of infecting the herd by implementing enhanced biosecurity plans.
  - Daily routine biosecurity has value for endemic disease (eg, brucellosis, tuberculosis, trichomoniasis, bovine viral diarrhea) but must be enhanced for FMD because the virus is so highly contagious and the US cattle herd lacks immunity.
  - The SBS Plan has resources for producers and their veterinarians to develop enhanced biosecurity plans before an outbreak based on the known exposure routes for FMD. Biosecurity checklists for feedlots and cattle on pasture, information manuals, templates, and biosecurity posters are available on the SBS Web site at: www.securebeef.org
- Include contingencies for periods of animal and animal product movement restrictions off of or onto the operation.
  - Contingency plans for holding cattle in place on operations (eg, farms, ranches, feedlots, livestock markets) and providing sufficient feed, water, and other husbandry needs will be necessary. Veterinarians can advise on options to ensure animal well-being during these times.
  - Veterinarians should also review state response plans for stopping cattle in transit (between production systems or to harvest) and discuss this with their clients.
- Align with state and federal guidelines to meet movement permit requirements when restrictions are lifted (see later discussion).

- Optimize the ability to quickly recognize and promptly report clinical signs in cattle.
  - Accredited veterinarians may be involved in sample collection, farm inspections, and teaching on-farm observers to recognize abnormal production parameters or clinical signs that may indicate early FMD.
    - Particularly for FMD, active observational surveillance may need to be routinely performed and documented to provide evidence of no infection. The *SBS Plan: Active Observational Surveillance for Foot and Mouth Disease: An Overview*, June 2017, is available at http://securebeef.org/Assets/SBS_Active-Observational-Surveillance-Overview.pdf.
    - Training materials, including videos for conducting surveillance and an FMD *Pocket Guide for Cattle*, with pictures of lesions, can be found on the SBS Web site at: www.securebeef.org.

These principles are also useful for other FADs and veterinarians should sit down with beef producer clients and use these resources to prepare now because

- Producers who worked with their veterinarian to implement routine endemic disease biosecurity protocols, and wrote enhanced biosecurity and business continuity plans ahead of time, are better positioned to request a movement permit.
- Producers who were trained by their veterinarian before an outbreak will be able to implement observational surveillance on the first day of an outbreak.
- Producers who are prepared to provide evidence of no disease and keep accurate records of all cattle movements may be more likely to receive a movement permit.

### *Preparing Veterinary Practices: Business Continuity Planning*

Veterinarians should also be aware of business continuity issues for their practices, including personnel and resources management. Although many veterinarians are familiar with the disruptions caused by incidences of endemic diseases with regulatory or reporting consequences (eg, tuberculosis, brucellosis, vesicular stomatitis), an FAD incursion (eg, bovine spongiform encephalopathy [BSE]; New World screwworm; and, in particular, FMD) would severely affect the ongoing operations of livestock-oriented veterinary practices. Practice owners should

- Develop contingency plans in the event the veterinarian is involved in an FAD investigation. For biosecurity reasons, it is best for that individual to refrain from other farm visits or contacting animals until additional precautions can be implemented.
- Develop contingencies if an animal within the clinic tests positive or if the practice is within a regulatory control area.
- Develop an enhanced biosecurity plan for the practice, including personnel and resource management, which prevents transmission from one farm to another.

For example, cattle shed FMD virus before any clinical signs are present, so all herds should be treated as potentially positive and strict cleaning and disinfection should be practiced between farms.

Some enhanced biosecurity recommendations for preventing FMD exposure include[12]

- Arriving at the cattle operation having showered, wearing clean clothing, and footwear since last contacting susceptible animals.

- All vehicles and equipment should be cleaned and effectively disinfected before entering the premises, otherwise entry is prohibited.
- Articles that are difficult to disinfect, such as halters or ropes, should not be transferred between operations but left at each farm for use on site.

### Preparing the Community: Involvement in Local and State Planning

The survival of the livestock or mixed animal veterinary practice is associated with the survival of the local livestock producers and industries. Providing preparedness advice to local producers and to the industry as a whole is critical to the business continuity of both the livestock industry and livestock veterinarians. Training and staying current is key to this, as is being actively involved in local and state preparedness and response planning.

Using USDA's FAD PReP guidance, multiple states have begun developing state-specific FAD plans and many seek input from industry and the private sector. Veterinarians should be aware of the USDA FAD PReP guidance and be knowledgeable of the response plans for the state or states in which they practice. Get involved through local organized veterinary and cattle associations to be part of the process. Response plans tend to be dynamic and input from veterinarians is sought during development and after release.

### RESPONDING TO A FOREIGN ANIMAL DISEASE OUTBREAK

The USDA FAD PReP critical activities to control and eradicate FADs and a few specific to FMD are listed in **Box 1**.[13] These critical activities and others will be carried out by the regulatory officials managing the outbreak in control areas set up around FMD-infected premises. Veterinary practitioners may be involved in helping accomplish several of these actions.

### Quarantine and Movement Controls

Animal and animal product movement will be prohibited from premises with infected animals,[14] and from premises with susceptible species located in the disease control area established by regulatory authorities (**Fig. 1**). Duration will vary depending on the specific outbreak:

- Any movement of susceptible species will be done via permit for specific movements (see later discussion). An FAD quarantine and movement control overview[15] is available at: http://www.cfsph.iastate.edu/pdf/fad-prep-nahems-tactical-topics-quarantine-movement-control.
- The size of the control area depends on the FAD of concern, characteristics of the infected premises, physical boundaries, jurisdictional areas, and other factors.[16]
- Livestock shipments already in transit at the time of the disease announcement will need to be directed to an acceptable destination for holding and observation.[17]
- More details about the type of movement as it relates to the premises designation and the control area can be found in the USDA *FAD Response Ready Reference Guide, Movement Control in an FAD Outbreak*, December 2015, available at: https://www.aphis.usda.gov/animal_health/emergency_management/downloads/fad_rrg_movement_control.pdf.

#### Movement permits and certificates of veterinary inspection

During the initial phases of an FMD outbreak, a stop movement order will be instituted and could be in place for some time. Once the outbreak extent is defined, a plan for

---

**Box 1**
**Select critical activities for a foot-and-mouth disease response**

Quarantine and movement controls

Biosecurity measures

Epidemiologic investigation and tracing

Increased surveillance

Continuity of business measures for noninfected and noncontaminated animal products

Mass depopulation and euthanasia (as response indicates)

Carcass disposal (as response indicates)

Emergency vaccination (as response indicates)

*Data from* USDA FAD PReP, FMD Response Plan, September 2014. Available at: https://www.aphis.usda.gov/animal_health/emergency_management/downloads/fmd_responseplan.pdf. Accessed November 28, 2017.

---

restarting movement of cattle with no evidence of infection that allows as much continuity of business as possible while minimizing the risk of FMD transmission will be implemented. Movement into, within, or from a control area will be by permit only and based on the risk posed by the item moved.[13] Movement permits facilitate

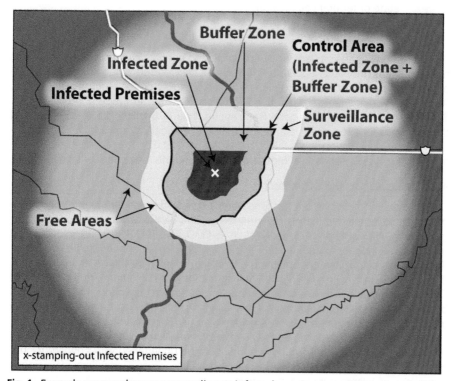

**Fig. 1.** Example areas and zones surrounding an infected premises in an FMD outbreak. (*From* USDA foot-and-mouth disease response plan, the red book. 2014. Available at: https://www.aphis.usda.gov/animal_health/emergency_management/downloads/fmd_responseplan.pdf. Accessed November 28, 2017; with permission.)

tracking of shipments and animals, and are issued by the officials managing the incident. Animal movements not associated with control areas will still require a Certificate of Veterinary Inspection (CVI) signed by an accredited veterinarian, and may be subject to additional requirements as defined by the receiving state; the role of CVIs for movement within a control area is being discussed among federal and state animal health officials; no official guidance is currently available.

Producers seeking movement permits will need to meet state and federal guidelines and veterinarians are a logical conduit for this information. Requirements for movement permits for premises within the control area may include

- Having a PIN
- Implementing biosecurity measures to control risk of disease entering or leaving the operation
- Providing epidemiologic information regarding all cattle movements and potential exposures
  - Keeping records of movement of animals, supplies, equipment, and people can provide accurate information about potential, or lack of, exposure risk (example movement logs are available on the SBS Web site at: www.securebeef.org)
- Conducting surveillance to demonstrate a lack of evidence of FMD infection
  - Negative diagnostic tests will likely be required before moving animals
    - Initially, and in a small outbreak, diagnostic samples may be collected by state or federal veterinarians
    - In a more extensive or prolonged FMD outbreak, private veterinarians may be needed and authorized to collect samples for testing.

FMD will present producers with unprecedented economic viability challenges and restarting cattle movement could be viewed as a lifeline to surviving an outbreak. Veterinarians may feel pressured to sign off on shipments that have not met all criteria. Accredited veterinarians are obligated to follow all state and federal requirements. This includes the Code of Federal Regulations, Title 9, Section 161.4, containing all the standards for accredited veterinarian duties, specifically (f), (g), and (h) for, respectively, reporting suspect cases, taking measures of sanitation to prevent spread of disease, and staying informed on regulations governing the movement of animals.[18]

### Mass Depopulation and Euthanasia

Depopulation or stamping out has long been a standard procedure to control FAD incursions and is included in the USDA response plan, particularly for small or focal outbreaks of highly contagious diseases such as FMD. The FAD PReP has guidelines for mass depopulation and euthanasia. Also, the American Veterinary Medical Association is developing mass depopulation guidelines to enhance their euthanasia materials.[19] (See Jan K. Shearer and colleagues' article, "Humane Euthanasia and Carcass Disposal," in this issue.) Veterinary practitioners may choose to be involved but will not be required to depopulate their client's cattle. This will be handled by those managing the outbreak and first responders.

Mass cattle depopulation in an FAD outbreak is challenging logistically and from an animal welfare standpoint. Depopulation should be undertaken with concern for human safety, animal welfare, and proper disposal of carcasses. Particularly for livestock operations with large numbers of animals on a site, such as large feedlots, depopulation is difficult and may not be feasible in an acceptable time frame for effective disease control.[20] This challenge also exists when outbreaks are geographically extensive in areas with high populations of FMD-susceptible species.

*Management of infected premises*

If the officials managing the outbreak determine depopulation is not warranted, numerous factors must be considered for managing the cattle through the outbreak. Veterinarians may be involved in helping clients implement plans to address the following critical factors:

- Enhancing biocontainment to prevent transmission offsite: Maintaining an infected premises through an outbreak is a substantial risk for disease transmission. All aspects of management will need strict control to minimize risk. Equipment, personnel, feed delivery, manure, wastewater, wildlife contact, and dust generation will all need to be controlled.
- Managing FMD morbidity: Most cattle on the operation will likely become infected and show some level of clinical signs. Providing support through feed and water and symptomatic treatment consistent with good animal welfare may be a substantial labor demand. Veterinarians can help their clients plan for humane euthanasia and disposal of severe cases.[21]
- Permitting cattle without clinical signs to move to harvest: This may occur when the movement to harvest can be made with minimal risk by implementing truck and driver biosecurity, and the feedlot and slaughter facility are in the same control area. As with any disease, the USDA Food Safety Inspection Service will not allow slaughter of animals with clinical signs.
- Limiting interaction of infected and noninfected cattle and fomites: Mixing of cattle in hospital facilities, or movement of personnel and equipment between pens or premises for treatments, may increase transmission within the feedlot or operation. Careful segregation of the feedlot into infected and noninfected areas may slow transmission and allow better allocation of labor resources. Alternately, if the labor demands of treating morbid cattle can be met, rapid transmission of disease through the feedlot may allow for a quicker outbreak. The sooner the outbreak can run through the all the cattle, the sooner the feedlot can begin to recover.

## Carcass Disposal

Carcass disposal in an FAD outbreak will be directed by the state and federal animal health officials managing the outbreak, ensuring all local, state, and federal regulations are met. Biosecurity measures are imperative if carcasses are moved to other locations for burial, composting, rendering, or alternative methods. APHIS, the Department of Homeland Security, the National Renderers Association, and other stakeholders are closely examining appropriate carcass disposal options for a US FMD outbreak. (See Jan K. Shearer and colleagues' article, "Humane Euthanasia and Carcass Disposal," in this issue.) Veterinary practitioners may choose to be involved but will not be required to help dispose of their client's cattle. This will be handled by those managing the outbreak and first responders.

At the time of this writing, federal carcass disposal regulations exist only for the cattle FAD, classic BSE. Veterinarians should already be aware of the US Food and Drug Administration regulations for mammalian protein used in ruminant feed, specifically regarding the disposition of animal carcasses from cattle older than 30 months of age, and tallow from, or animals with, BSE.[22–25] Also, the Environmental Protection Agency considers the prion infectious agent a pest under the Federal Insecticide, Fungicide, and Rodenticide Act, and, as such, considers "prions to be a form of plant or animal life which is injurious to health or the environment." Information is available at: https://www.epa.gov/sites/production/files/2015-09/documents/records_of_

decision_on_prions.pdf. BSE case investigations are federally regulated by APHIS and the agency currently considers the use of alkaline hydrolysis tissue digesters as the preferred method of disposal for BSE contaminated carcasses.[26]

### Emergency Vaccination

There are currently no specific federal protocols or policies for the use of vaccination for US cattle FADs. APHIS has some guidance for the use of vaccination during an FMD event in the US, yet several details remain to be determined. As written, APHIS and the SAHOs, with input from industry, will decide on the use of vaccination in an FMD event.[27] There will be differences among states given their respective resources, infrastructure, and industry structures (eg, cow-calf, feeders, small and large dairies); and state response plans may include vaccination plans. Specific details describing the private veterinarians' role in the vaccine delivery has not been finalized. Depending on the size and scope of outbreak, it is likely that private veterinarians will be included in the vaccination campaign. The use of trained laypeople, such as feedyard personnel, with veterinary oversight, might also be used in the event of a large or extended outbreak. Implementing FMD vaccination will be a massive undertaking and veterinarians will be essential in its effective implementation. All involved will be required to accurately document the chain of custody for the vaccine, properly handle and store it, and document delivery to each individual animal. Veterinarians should familiarize themselves with their state's response plan and the APHIS decisions regarding FMD vaccination programs.

## COMMUNICATION

Veterinarians serve as a trusted resource for their clients and the public and should stay informed in the event of a US FAD outbreak. A reliable resource for FMD information is www.FootAndMouthDiseaseInfo.org, which was developed by the national livestock industry FMD Cross-Species Team, representing beef, pork, dairy, and sheep. The beef industry developed a similar informational Web site during the 2003 BSE case.

Consistent messaging of basic disease facts from industry, veterinarians, and state and federal animal health authorities provides accurate information to the public, minimizes fear of the unknown, and provides positive impacts to the negative market implications during an FAD event. In an FMD outbreak, veterinarians can remind clients and consumer that FMD is not a public health or food safety concern. Meat and milk are safe to eat and drink.

## SUMMARY

Private practice veterinarians are a tremendous resource for their clients and local community when preparing for and responding to an FAD outbreak. It is important for veterinarians to stay current on clinical signs and syndromes suggestive of FADs. Encouraging clients to call when cattle are off or unusual signs are observed, and reaching out to state and federal animal health officials can make the difference between a widespread outbreak and rapid containment.

Numerous resources exist for veterinarians to train themselves about animal health emergencies, and help their clients prepare and develop business continuity plans. The success of veterinary practices is closely tied to the livelihood of their clients. Time spent preparing clients is time well spent.

As trusted advisors, clients will turn to veterinarians in times of need. Lead by example and ensure the veterinary practice has a business continuity plan. An FAD outbreak will require a concerted effort by producers, veterinarians, emergency responders, and state and federal officials to successfully control and eradicate the disease. Be part of the success; start preparing today.

**REFERENCES**

1. South Sudan livestock crisis. Food and Agriculture Organization of the United Nations. 2015. Available at: http://www.fao.org/fileadmin/user_upload/emergencies/docs/FAOSS%20Livestock%20Crisis%20Update%202015.pdf. Accessed November 28, 2017.
2. Tuppurainen ES, Oura CA. Review: lumpy skin disease: an emerging threat to Europe, the Middle East and Asia. Transbound Emerg Dis 2012;59(1):40–8.
3. USDA-AHPIS VS. APHIS foreign animal disease framework, roles and coordination. 2016. Available at: https://www.aphis.usda.gov/animal_health/emergency_management/downloads/documents_manuals/fadprep_manual_1.pdf. Accessed November 28, 2017.
4. USDA-APHIS VS. The imperative for foreign animal disease preparedness and response. 2016. Available at: https://www.aphis.usda.gov/animal_health/emergency_management/downloads/intro_fadprep.pdf. Accessed November 28, 2017.
5. Clifford J. Hearing to review the advances of animal health within the livestock industry. 110th Congress. House of Representatives, Committee on Agriculture. 2008.
6. USDA-APHIS VS. Calendar year 2016 update: FAD Investigation report. 2017. Available at: https://www.aphis.usda.gov/animal_health/emergency_management/downloads/summary_fad_investigations.pdf. Accessed November 28, 2017.
7. National Incident Management System. Federal Emergency Management Agency. 2017. Available at: https://www.fema.gov/national-incident-management-system. Accessed November 28, 2017.
8. Taylor TK, Flaming KP, Bickett-Weddle DA, et al. 2015 USDA National Veterinary Accreditation Program Module 19: animal health emergency response. Available at: https://www.aphis.usda.gov/aphis/ourfocus/animalhealth/nvap/ct_aast. Accessed November 28, 2017.
9. McReynolds SM, Sanderson MW, Reeves A, et al. Modeling the impact of vaccination control strategies of a foot and mouth disease outbreak in the Central United States. Prev Vet Med 2014;117:487–504.
10. Infection with foot and mouth disease virus. OIE Terrestrial Animal Health Code. 2017. Available at: http://www.oie.int/index.php?id=169&L=0&htmfile=chapitre_fmd.htm. Accessed November 28, 2017.
11. Bickett-Weddle DA, Dewell RD, Obbink K, et al. The planned response to an FMD outbreak is not what it used to be. In: Bovine practitioner, Annual Meeting of the American Association of Bovine Practitioners. 2017.
12. Self-Assessment checklist for enhanced biosecurity for FMD prevention. Secure beef supply. 2017. Available at: www.securebeef.org/ beef-producers/biosecurity/. Accessed November 28, 2017.
13. USDA Foot-and-Mouth Disease Response Plan, The Red Book. September 2014. Available at: https://www.aphis.usda.gov/animal_health/emergency_management/downloads/fmd_responseplan.pdf. Accessed on November 28, 2017.
14. USDA-APHIS VS. FAD PReP permitted movement. 2017. Available at: https://www.aphis.usda.gov/animal_health/emergency_management/downloads/documents_manuals/fadprep_man6-0_permit-mvmt.pdf. Accessed November 28, 2017.

15. Center for Food Security and Public Health. FAD PReP/NAHEMS Tactical topics: quarantine and movement control. 2017. Available at: http://www.cfsph.iastate.edu/pdf/fad-prep-nahems-tactical-topics-quarantine-movement-control. Accessed November 28, 2017.
16. USDA-APHIS VS Preparedness and Incident Coordination. National center for animal health emergency management: zones, areas, and premises designations in a foreign animal disease outbreak. Available at: https://www.aphis.usda.gov/animal_health/emergency_management/downloads/premises_and_zones.pdf. Accessed November 28, 2017.
17. Managed movement of cattle in the U.S. in a foot and mouth disease outbreak. Secure beef supply plan. 2016. Available at: http://securebeef.org/Assets/SBS_Managed-Movement_DRAFT.pdf. Accessed November 28, 2017.
18. Title 9 Animals and Animal Products, Volume 1, Section 161.4 Standards for accredited veterinarian duties. Code of Federal Regulations. 2017. Available at: https://www.law.cornell.edu/cfr/text/9/161.4. Accessed November 28, 2017.
19. Center for Food Security and Public Health, USDA. FAD PReP NAHEMS guidelines: mass depopulation and euthanasia. 2015. Available at: http://www.cfsph.iastate.edu/pdf/fad-prep-nahems-guidelines-mass-depopulation-and-euthanasia. Accessed November 28, 2017.
20. McReynolds SM, Sanderson MW. Feasibility of depopulation of a large feedlot during a foot-and-mouth disease outbreak. J Am Vet Med Assoc 2014;244:291–8.
21. BQA, IVMA, Iowa Beef Center. Caring for compromised cattle. Available at: https://bqa.unl.edu/documents/Caring%20for%20Compromised%20Cattle.pdf. Accessed November 28, 2017.
22. Substances prohibited from use in animal food or feed, effective April 27, 2009, regarding use of carcasses from cattle 30 months of age and older and carcasses/tallow from BSE positive cattle. 21 CFR Part 589. Available at: https://www.fda.gov/animalveterinary/guidancecomplianceenforcement/complianceenforcement/bovinespongiformencephalopathy/ucm115754.htm. Accessed November 28, 2017.
23. Bovine spongiform encephalopathy. Food and Drug Administration. 2017. Available at: https://www.fda.gov/AnimalVeterinary/GuidanceComplianceEnforcement/ComplianceEnforcement/BovineSpongiformEncephalopathy/default.htm. Accessed November 28, 2017.
24. Feed ban enhancement: implementation questions and answers. Food and Drug Administration. 2017. Available at: https://www.fda.gov/AnimalVeterinary/GuidanceComplianceEnforcement/ComplianceEnforcement/BovineSpongiformEncephalopathy/ucm114453.htm. Accessed November 28, 2017.
25. USDA-APHIS VS. About BSE. 2016. Available at: https://www.aphis.usda.gov/aphis/ourfocus/animalhealth/animal-disease-information/cattle-disease-information/sa_bse/ct_about_bse. Accessed November 28, 2017.
26. USDA-APHIS VS. FAD PReP NAHEMS operational guidelines: disposal. 2005. Available at: https://www.aphis.usda.gov/emergency_response/tools/on-site/htdocs/images/nahems_disposal.pdf. Accessed November 28, 2017.
27. Center for Food Security and Public Health, USDA. FAD Prep NAHEMS: vaccination for contagious diseases appendix a: foot and mouth disease. 2015. Available at: http://www.cfsph.iastate.edu/pdf/fad-prep-nahems-appendix-a-vaccination-for-foot-and-mouth-disease. Accessed November 28, 2017.

# Humane Euthanasia and Carcass Disposal

Jan K. Shearer, DVM, MS[a],*, Dee Griffin, DVM, MS[b], Scott E. Cotton, MS, CPRM[c]

## KEYWORDS

- Bovine • Euthanasia • Humane • Carcass disposal • Composting • Rendering
- Burial • Incineration

## KEY POINTS

- Effective euthanasia depends on selection of the appropriate firearm, bullet or shotshell, and use of the proper anatomic site.
- Unlike euthanasia with a firearm, captive bolt requires animal restraint for close contact with the animal and accurate placement of the device over the proper anatomic site.
- It is critical to have disaster carcass disposal plans in place at the state and county levels that are reviewed regularly; these plans must involve both the state's environmental control agency and the state's animal industry agency.
- There are 7 methods of beef carcass disposal: packing plant slaughter, rendering, composting, burial, incineration, open burning and, in the future, mobile hydrothermal carbonization units.
- Disposal method selection is influenced by state/federal targeted disease control, such as foreign animal disease; the number of cattle involved in the disaster incident; the opportunity to delay, stagger, or prolong the disposal; the environmental fragility at the incident location; the climate at the time of the incident; the materials available to be used in association with the disposal; the available equipment needed to manage the carcasses; and political-social-regulatory pressures.

## INTRODUCTION

Euthanasia is ending life in a way that minimizes or eliminates pain and distress. It requires techniques that induce an immediate loss of consciousness followed by cardiac and respiratory arrest and, ultimately, a cessation of brain function. On the contrary, killing is the ending of life in a way that does not meet the definition of euthanasia. Some degree of pain and distress is unavoidable because the transition from

Disclosure Statement: The authors have nothing to disclose.

[a] Department of Veterinary Diagnostic and Production Animal Medicine, College of Veterinary Medicine, Iowa State University, 2436 Lloyd Veterinary Medical Center, Ames, IA 50011, USA; [b] Texas A&M Veterinary Medical Center, West Texas A&M University, Box 60998, Canyon, TX 79016-0001, USA; [c] University of Wyoming Extension, 2011 Fairgrounds Road, Casper, WY 82604, USA

* Corresponding author.

*E-mail address:* jks@iastate.edu

consciousness to unconsciousness is delayed. Euthanasia is the objective when it is necessary to relieve uncontrollable animal suffering, but it is not always possible. For example, recent wildfires in the Midwest and flooding associated with hurricanes in Texas, Louisiana, and Florida left cattle stranded in extreme misery, without food or drinkable water. Rather than compound their distress by attempting to gather these animals or simply allow them to linger and suffer for days or weeks before death, for the sake of the animals' welfare, people opted to end their misery in the most expedient way possible. Such conditions often preclude targeting anatomic sites on the skull that would assure immediate loss of consciousness. Unpleasant as it is, humans have a moral responsibility to act in the best interests of animals in situations that may require ending their life, keeping in mind that no one is absolved of the obligation to use the most humane methods available whenever possible.[1] Euthanasia may also be justified when there is no obvious injury but the ability to rescue animals from unlivable conditions is not possible. Consider an animal that falls into a sinkhole that cannot be extricated or cattle stranded in flooded lowlands after a hurricane. Surrounded by brackish water and unable to be moved, in stifling heat and humidity with no available pasture or way to hydrate themselves, cattle are likely to die a slow and miserable death. Euthanasia in these circumstances may be the only option to relieve suffering.

Federal, state, and local laws regulate carcass disposal. Where euthanasia of animals has been conducted using barbiturates or barbituric acid derivatives, the persistence of drug residues poses risks for scavenging wildlife and adulteration of rendered products used for animal feed. Open pyre burning of carcass remains is not permitted in many states and most landfills do not accept livestock mortalities. Disposal methods for consideration in disaster situations include packing plant slaughter, rendering, composting, burial, incineration, open burning, and hydrothermal carbonization. Selection of the most appropriate method depends on the number of carcasses requiring disposal, potential environmental impact, climatic conditions, and many other factors. Preplanning and training are key requirements for the proper application of euthanasia procedures and disposal of carcasses.

## METHODS OF EUTHANASIA

Conditions and/or venues that may require euthanasia vary greatly; therefore, veterinarians should be prepared to conduct the procedure using the method most appropriate for the situation.[1]

### Injectable Anesthetics

Barbiturates and barbituric acid derivative anesthetic-type agents are often preferred because of their rapid action and ability to induce a smooth transition from consciousness to unconsciousness and death. Drawbacks to the use of these agents for euthanasia include cost, the need for restraint to deliver the drug, necessity to maintain a careful accounting of amounts used, regulatory requirements that specify these agents be administered only by a veterinarian, and residues that may limit carcass disposal options. In situations requiring euthanasia of numerous animals, it may difficult to secure a sufficient amount of the drug to meet euthanasia needs. For these reasons, barbiturates are not likely the ideal choice for conducting euthanasia in disaster situations.

### Firearms

Firearms are the most common method used for on-farm euthanasia of cattle.[2] Death is caused by massive destruction of brain tissue. Despite its popularity and effectiveness for the purpose of euthanasia, those who are less familiar with firearms often find gunshot violent and objectionable. When properly conducted, however, euthanasia by gunshot is humane.

### Specific recommendations on firearms for euthanasia

Most important is the selection of the most appropriate caliber and bullet or shotshell for size and age of the animal to be euthanized. Handguns or pistols are short-barreled firearms that may be fired with 1 hand. For the purposes of euthanasia, handguns are limited to close-range shooting (within 2–3 ft [61–91 cm]) of the intended target. Calibers ranging from .32 to .45 are recommended for euthanasia of adult cattle, sheep, and swine.[3] Solid-point lead bullets are recommended over hollow-point bullets because they are more likely to traverse the skull. Hollow-point bullets are designed to expand and fragment on impact with their targets, which reduces the depth of penetration. The bullet from a .22 caliber handgun is unable to achieve desirable muzzle energy and is, therefore, not recommended for euthanasia of adult cattle, large boars or sows, and horned rams regardless of the type of bullet used.[4,5]

Rifles are long-barreled firearms normally fired from the shoulder. They are preferred for euthanasia when it is necessary to shoot from a distance. Rifles are capable of delivering projectiles at a much higher muzzle velocities compared with handguns. Higher muzzle velocities increase the pounds of force or energy bullets dispense to their targets on impact. From a safety perspective, this is important because the use of higher-caliber firearms increases the possibility that a bullet passes through its target thus posing a danger to bystanders. On the contrary, bullets fired from lower-caliber firearms have decreased muzzle velocity and reduced force that may be insufficient to penetrate the skull. It is for this reason that the .22 long rifle is not recommended as a firearm for routine euthanasia in cattle.[4,5] General recommendations on rifle selection for euthanasia of adult cattle, sheep, and swine include .22 magnum, .223, .243, and .270, among others. Similar to the recommendations for use of handguns, at close range and firing at the skull, a solid-point bullet is preferred because maximum penetration of the bullet is desired. When necessary to fire from a distance and the target is the heart/lungs of the thorax, a hollow-point bullet may be preferred because fragmentation and expansion of the bullet increases damage at the impact site, which is more desirable at this anatomic site.[1]

Shotguns loaded with buckshot or shotshells (BB shot) are appropriate from a distance of 1 yd to 2 yd (.9–1.8 m). Some people prefer to use shotgun slugs. At close range, shotgun slugs are generally unnecessary. Whenever shooting from a distance, however, shotgun slugs are preferred over BB shot. The preferred gauges for euthanasia of mature cattle, large boars, and rams are 20, 16, and 12 gauges if BB shot is used and slugs if a 28 or .410 gauge is used.[1] General recommendations/suggestions on firearm and ammunition selection for euthanasia of calves and young animals as well as of adult cows and bulls are listed in **Table 1**.

### Safety considerations with use of firearms for euthanasia

The drawback to gunshot as a method of euthanasia is danger for those who are unfamiliar with firearms. Aside from the possibility of unintentionally shooting oneself or a bystander by misdirection of the muzzle, anything that might obstruct or occlude the muzzle could cause the barrel to explode, resulting in great danger for the shooter and anyone nearby. For safety reasons it is important that the muzzle of a shotgun (or any other firearm) never be held directly against an animal's head. Discharge of a firearm results in the development of enormous pressure within the barrel. If either the muzzle

**Table 1**
**General recommendations on firearm and ammunition selections for euthanasia of cattle**

|  | Handguns | Rifles | Shotguns |
| --- | --- | --- | --- |
| Calves/young animals | .32 or larger caliber Solid-point bullet (within 2–3 ft) | .22 long rifle or larger caliber Solid-point bullet (at close range) | .410–20 gauge 4–6 birdshot or buckshot (within 3–6 ft) |
| Adult cattle | .32–.45 caliber Solid-point bullet (within 2–3 ft) | .22 magnum or higher caliber Solid-point bullet (at close range) | 20–12 gauge Buckshot or slug (within 3–6 ft) |
| Mature bulls | .38–.45 caliber Solid-point bullet (within 2–3 ft) | .22 magnum or higher caliber Solid-point bullet (at close range) | 20–12 gauge Buckshot or slug (within 3–6 ft) |

or the barrel is obstructed, the barrel is likely to explode causing great risk to the shooter and others.

Firearms are noisy; therefore, ear protection is advised for the shooter and by-standers. This may be somewhat less of a problem outdoors; but inside a building, the noise from a firearm can be disturbing not only for animals but also for coworkers. Noise suppressors (silencers or noise reducers) can be legally fitted to the muzzle of guns in most states. The regulations for purchasing a suppressor are similar to those required for the purchasing a firearm (**Box 1**).

## CONSIDERATIONS FOR EUTHANASIA OF AMBULATORY ANIMALS

The ability to get within close range of nonambulatory and weak or debilitated animals permits less difficulty for conducting euthanasia procedures. On the contrary, animals that are mobile and potentially fractious may provide significant challenges for proper application of euthanasia procedures because animals may need to be shot from some distance. If possible, the containment of animals to a suitable area with a safe background for use of firearms is best. Ideally, the distance between the technician and the target animal should be no more than 20 yd. At distances beyond 25 yd, most professional shooters start to have a high percentages of misses. At distances greater than 50 yd, fewer than 10% of professional shooters are accurate.

**Box 1**
**Safety considerations for firearm use**

1. Always treat firearms as though they are loaded.
2. Always be sure that the firearm is pointed in a safe direction.
3. Avoid contact with the trigger until you are ready to fire.
4. Be sure of your target and what is beyond it.
5. Keep bystanders a safe distance behind the shooter at all times.
6. Be sure you are familiar with the firearm and how it functions.
7. To avoid possible explosion of the barrel, never hold the muzzle of a firearm flush against the skull.

Fatigue sets in when targeting technicians expend more than 200 rounds. After the first 100 rounds, there is often a 10% to 15% increase in misses. When large numbers of animals must be euthanized, it is important to have enough shooters to prevent poor marksmanship that might result from fatigue.

## CAPTIVE BOLT

Captive bolt (CB) is a popular method of euthanasia for livestock in field situations. Penetrating CB is generally required for adult animals in on-farm settings; however, either penetrating or nonpenetrating CB is suitable for euthanasia of young animals. Whether used in mature or young animals, it is highly recommended that an adjunctive method (secondary step) be used in conjunction with CB to assure death. A recent study in cattle by Gilliam and colleagues[6] found that death occurred approximately 90% of the time without the use of a secondary adjunctive step. Approximately 10% of animals re-established a pattern of rhythmic breathing and other indicators suggestive of a possible return to consciousness. Based on these data, American Veterinary Medical Association (AVMA) guidelines[1] and the authors strongly suggest use of a secondary step to assure death.

Styles of penetrating CB include an in-line (cylindrical) and pistol grip (resembling a handgun) versions (**Fig. 1**). Pneumatic CB guns (air powered) are primarily limited to use in slaughter plant environments. Models using gunpowder charges are more often used in farm environments. Depending on model, the bolt may automatically retract or require manual placement back into the barrel through the muzzle.

Accurate placement of the CB over the ideal anatomic site, bolt velocity, and depth of penetration determine effectiveness of a device's ability to cause a loss of consciousness and death. Bolt velocity is dependent on maintenance, in particular cleaning of the CB and proper storage of the cartridge charges. CB guns should be cleaned regularly using the same or similar solvents used in the cleaning of firearms. Powder charges for CB guns should be stored in airtight containers to prevent absorption of moisture, which may result in soft shots (ie, reduced bolt velocity). Nonpenetrating CB guns should not be used for the euthanasia of adult cattle, sheep, or swine. It is appropriate for euthanasia of young animals when followed by the use of an adjunctive (secondary step) method to assure death. An important difference between the use of CB and firearms is that restraint is often required to place the muzzle of the CB in direct

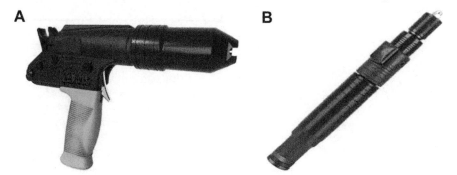

**Fig. 1.** Penetrating CB stunners. (*A*) Jarvis .25 caliber long bolt (pistol grip design) penetrating CB stunner. (*Courtesy of* Jarvis Products Corp, Middletown, CT; with permission.) and (*B*) Schermer KR in-line penetrating CB (*B*). (*Courtesy of* Koch Supplies, North Kansas City, MO; and Karl Schermer GmbH & Co. KG, Ettlingen, Germany.)

contact with the skull over the intended anatomic site. Once the device is in place, discharge of the CB should occur with little or no delay so that animal distress is minimized.

## ADJUNCTIVE (SECONDARY) METHODS TO ASSURE DEATH

Adjunctive methods to assure death should be applied immediately after (never before) an animal is determined to be unconscious. The most common methods are pithing, exsanguination, intravenous injection of a salt solution (ie, saturated solution of potassium chloride or magnesium sulfate), and second or third shot. None of these secondary methods prevents rendering or interferes with other carcass disposal methods.

Pithing involves the insertion of a flexible rod or wire through the hole in the skull produced by the bolt of the penetrative CB (**Fig. 2**). Once the pithing rod enters the cranial cavity, it is directed toward the brainstem and spinal cord. The pithing rod should be manipulated in a back-and-forth manner to cause maximum damage to brainstem tissues. Bystanders are advised to stand clear of feet and legs because most animals may exhibit violent involuntary muscle contraction during the pithing process.

Exsanguination is performed by severing major blood vessels arising to and from the heart. Death results from a precipitous drop in blood volume and pressure. Specifically, a sharp knife is directed into the jugular furrow of the neck and toward the thoracic inlet or chest to maximize blood flow from the carotid arteries and jugular veins. This assures a more rapid flow of blood and a shorter time to death (**Fig. 3**).

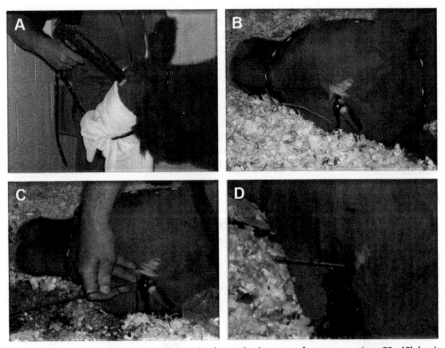

**Fig. 2.** Pithing procedure. (*A*) euthanasia through the use of a penetrating CB, (*B*) brain matter is visible protruding through the hole in the skull produced by the bolt, (*C*) a metal pithing rod is inserted into the hole in the skull and directed toward the brainstem where it is manipulated to maximize damage to brainstem tissues, and (*D*) pithing rod fully inserted through brainstem tissues into the spinal canal.

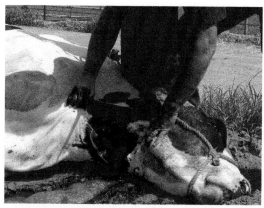

**Fig. 3.** Exsanguination is performed by directing a sharp knife into the jugular furrow cutting through the carotid arteries and jugular veins. Death results from low blood volume and pressure.

The intravenous administration of a saturated solution either of potassium chloride, magnesium chloride, or magnesium sulfate is recognized as an effective adjunctive step to assure death. Potassium chloride induces cardiac arrest, whereas magnesium salts cause death by suppression of neural activity.[1] Because they must be administered intravenously, these methods are less convenient for use in mass depopulation scenarios.

Finally, a second or third shot may also be used to assure death. The mechanism for causing death with a follow-up shot is simply to induce additional brain damage. When firearms are used, some people direct a bullet toward the heart as a possible second or third step. In all cases, the secondary or adjunctive step is applied only after it has been determined that the animal is unconscious.[1]

## VISUAL INDICATORS OF UNCONSCIOUSNESS

It is critically important to know the visual and clinical indicators of unconsciousness, because use of an adjunctive step to assure death causes great pain and distress in a conscious animal. Unconsciousness may be confirmed by noting the following: (1) if the animal is standing, it collapses immediately after the shot, initially appearing quite rigid for the first 20 seconds to 30 seconds after which time it gradually relaxes; (2) the animal may exhibit brief tetanic spasms and uncoordinated hind limb movements for several minutes in the postshot period, but at no time should there be any evidence of an attempt to rise or right itself; (3) there is an immediate and sustained cessation of rhythmic breathing; (4) there should be no vocalization, although on occasion there may be sounds associated with air being expelled through the upper respiratory tract; and (5) there are no corneal or palpebral reflexes present and eyes appear glazed or glassy with a dilated pupil.[7]

Immediately after the shot, check the corneal and palpebral reflexes. If these reflexes are absent, it is safe to apply one of the secondary steps to assure death. If an adjunctive step is not applied, it is essential to continue monitoring these visual and clinical signs until death is confirmed. Death as determined by cardiac arrest may require 7 minutes to 8 minutes or on occasion longer without the use of an adjunctive step.

## ANATOMIC LANDMARKS FOR EUTHANASIA OF LIVESTOCK

The objective in euthanasia is to cause sufficient damage to the brain to cause an immediate loss of consciousness resulting in death. This requires that the bullet or bolt damage vital structures. Proper anatomic site selection and aiming are key to the achievement of successful euthanasia (**Fig. 4**). Several methods may be used to determine the proper anatomic site for conducting euthanasia with either a firearm or CB (**Fig. 5**).

For cattle, the method published in the 2013 euthanasia guidelines recommends that the point of entry for a projectile be at the intersection of 2 imaginary lines, each drawn from the outside corner (lateral canthus) of the eye to the center of the base of the opposite horn.[1] This site is approximately 3 in (7.6 cm) anterior to the poll in a mature Holstein cow or approximately 2.5 in (6.35 cm) for a feedlot steer or heifer of 800 lb to 1200 lb (365 kg to 545 kg). The equivalent of this site may also be determined as half-way between 2 lines drawn laterally; 1 across the top of the poll and the other from lateral canthus to lateral canthus of the eyes.[8] Finally, a recent report describes the ideal point of entry as on the midline between the base of the ears at the level of the external acoustic meatus.[9]

The path of the trajectory should be approximately perpendicular to the anatomic sites described. Even when an animal is well restrained, however, slight or even significant variances in the angle of trajectory are possible. In a study of the euthanasia of sheep by CB, researchers observed that despite evidence of a consistent site of entry, the trajectory of the bolt and tissues disrupted by the bolt varied considerably.[10] The potential for variability is even greater when firearms are used. For example, the entry site for a projectile in an animal that is standing and facing a shooter is less likely to be perpendicular to the skull compared with an animal that is nonambulatory (ie, down in sternal recumbency) and facing a shooter who is standing above and looking downward.

## RESTRAINT TO IMPROVE SHOT ACCURACY AND SAFETY

The use of CB for euthanasia requires close contact with an animal because it is necessary to place the muzzle of the device flush with the skull over the intended site. For moribund animals, minimal restraint of the head with a halter is usually

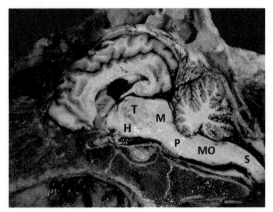

**Fig. 4.** Sagittal section of the bovine brain with key structures of the diencephalon including the thalamus (T) and hypothalamus (H), and the brainstem, which includes the midbrain (M), pons (P), and medulla oblongata (MO). Beyond the MO is the spinal cord (S).

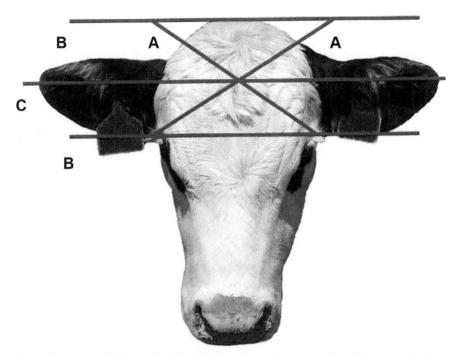

**Fig. 5.** The anatomic site may be identified as A, on the intersection of 2 lines each drawn from the lateral canthus of the eyes to the base of the opposite horn (ie, where the horn would be in a horned animal); B, on the midline of the skull midway between 2 horizontal lines—1 drawn between the lateral canthus of each eye and another drawn laterally across the poll; and C, on the midline between the base of the ears at the level of the external acoustic meatus.

sufficient. For fractious animals or those that are ambulatory, it may be necessary to use a firearm and follow-up with secondary steps as necessary. The temptation with animals that are mobile and potentially dangerous is to move them into a restraint chute where they can be safely restrained. The problem is to euthanize an animal in a chute risks significant difficulty in removal of the carcass from the chute. Chemical restraint using a tranquilizer, such as xylazine HCl, or a paralyzing agent, such as succinylcholine, is an option that may be considered in such situations. These may be administered to the animal while it is safely restrained in the chute. After delivery of the drug, the animal is released from the chute and monitored until such time that it may be safely approached and euthanized in a location where the carcass may be accessed by removal equipment. Note that xylazine HCl is an effective tranquilizer; but when animals are highly agitated or excited, its effectiveness in maintaining animals in tranquilized state is less predictable. The paralytic response to the administration of succinylcholine is more predictable and may provide safer conditions for follow-up euthanasia whether by CB or firearm. With the latter drug in particular, it is important that euthanasia be conducted as soon as possible after immobilization.

A final thought for those considering the use of succinylcholine or xylazine HCl: the inadvertent or accidental injection of either of these compounds into oneself or an assistant could be fatal. For this reason, it is highly recommended that these drugs be delivered by use of a pole syringe (even if given to an animal in a chute) to avoid inadvertent injection of oneself. Details and materials necessary for construction of a pole syringe are displayed in **Fig. 6**. Xylazine HCl and succinylcholine are effective at low doses in cattle. Xylazine is denatured at 165°C, which is well below rendering temperatures that are normally in excess of 240°C.

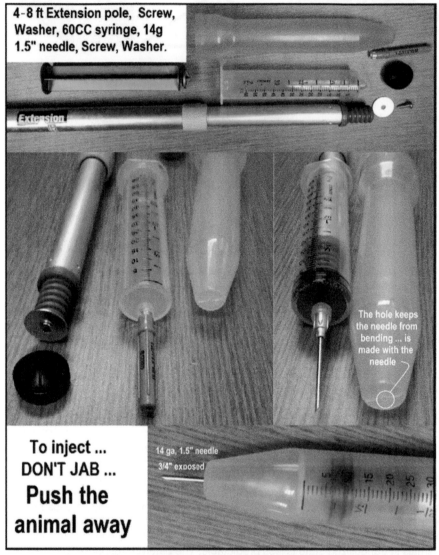

4-8 ft Extension pole, Screw, Washer, 60CC syringe, 14g 1.5" needle, Screw, Washer.

Extension

The hole keeps the needle from bending ... is made with the needle

To inject ...
DON'T JAB ...
Push the animal away

14 ga, 1.5" needle
3/4" exposed

**Fig. 6.** Components for construction of a pole syringe (produced by the author, D. Griffin). A pole syringe can be constructed using a small-diameter telescoping painter's pole that has had a washer attached to the end for accepting the black rubber seal from the plunger of a 60-mL disposable syringe. The painter's pole with attached 60-mL syringe becomes a tool for delivering a sedative/tranquilizer to the bovine. Note, it is best to use the largest injection needle available, such as a 14-gauge, 1.5 in. Additionally, it is useful to use the plastic syringe case with a needle size hole punched in the end to cover the syringe and needle. This covering helps prevent the injection needle from bending.

## UNACCEPTABLE METHODS

The methods of euthanasia deemed unacceptable include (1) manually applied blunt force trauma (as with a large hammer), (2) injection of chemical agents or other substances not specifically designed or labeled for euthanasia (disinfectants, cleaning solutions, and so forth), (3) air injection into the vein, (4) electrocution as with a 120-V electrical cord, (5) drowning, (6) exsanguination of conscious animals, and (7) deep tranquilization as with xylazine or other $\alpha_2$-agonist followed by potassium chloride or magnesium sulfate.[1] Although some people have been forced out of desperation to resort to 1 or more of these methods, readers are strongly advised against their use. Several of these methods are known to result in a less than humane death and for others the level of pain or distress associated with these methods is unknown. For example, use of xylazine to create a deep state of tranquilization followed by the rapid administration of potassium chloride is used by some veterinarians. The position of the AVMA is that this combination of agents should not be used for euthanasia. As stated in *Goodman and Gilman's The Pharmacologic Basis of Therapeutics*, 11th edition, "Although large doses of alpha-2 agonists can produce a state resembling general anesthesia, they are recognized as being unreliable for that purpose."[11] Results of an Iowa State University study confirm that even with extremely high doses of xylazine HCl, achievement of an anesthetic state is not possible.

## CONFIRMATION OF DEATH

Regardless of method used for conducting euthanasia procedures, it is important to confirm death, which is sometimes more easily said than done. The most reliable criteria include lack of pulse, breathing, corneal reflex, and response to firm toe pinch; inability to hear respiratory sounds and heart beat by use of a stethoscope; graying of the mucous membranes; and rigor mortis. None of these signs alone, with exception of rigor mortis, confirms death.[1]

## CARCASS DISPOSAL

Carcass disposal associated with foreign animal disease (FAD) is under the control of the United States Department of Agriculture (USDA) Animal and Plant Health Inspection Service (APHIS), Veterinary Services (VS), working in conjunction with state animal industry agencies. Carcass disposal information related to targeted diseases under the control of the USDA-APHIS is referred to the Foreign Animal Disease Preparedness and Response Plan of the USDA-APHIS-VS.[12]

It is critical for federal, state, and county agencies to have a carcass disposal plan in place to deal with livestock death disasters and for these groups to review these plans regularly with livestock producer and community groups. There are currently 7 methods of carcass disposal during a disaster: packing plant slaughter, rendering, composting, burial, incineration, open carcass burning, and mobile hydrothermal carbonization. The disposal methods selected are influenced by the number of cattle involved in the disaster incident; the opportunity to delay, stagger, or prolong the disposal; the environmental fragility at the incident location; climate considerations at the time of the incident; materials available to be used in association with the disposal; available equipment needed to manage the carcasses; and political-social-regulatory pressures.

## PLANNING FOR ANIMAL MORTALITY DISASTERS

Federal planning for livestock mortality disasters cannot account for the unique needs of individual states, counties, and communities. Therefore, state animal industry and environmental control agencies need to jointly develop contingency plans for addressing livestock mortality disasters. Planning should start as an outline that considers each state agency's mandated responsibilities to their associated federal agency. Plans should be assessed in regard to the needs and limitations within each state, county, and community within the country. For example, the southern coastal states present unique problems related to animal disposal associated with their climate (temperature, humidity, and precipitation) that are entirely different than high elevation desert states. Soil types and hydrology are critical in the deliberations if carcass burial or composting is considered. For example, the Texas Panhandle has more than 3 million cattle, low annual precipitation, and deep ground water. A casual assessment could lead to believing carcass burial might be an excellent option during a livestock mortality disaster, but soil scientist and hydrologist assessment indicates otherwise. Regardless of the area in the United States, site selection is the most important task in disaster mortality planning. Environmental soil engineers must be part of the planning team.

Besides site selection, planning must include an inventory of resources that can be mobilized in a livestock mortality emergency. For example, in concentrated livestock areas, rendering services are typically readily available and can be included as part of the carcass disposal plan, whereas in non–livestock-concentrated areas, rendering may have minimal role in the mortality disposal plan. Emergencies that do not involve immediate deaths, as is the case in an FAD, such as foot-and-mouth disease, mortalities under the control of the USDA-APHIS might be staggered, which could allow time to more efficiently use resources. Additionally, some disease emergencies do not threaten food safety and, therefore, harvesting or salvaging cattle at packers could allow staggered mortality control.

Too often initial planning is not followed-up with development of specific action plans. To avoid crisis action paralysis, cattle owners should gather a team (veterinarian, nutritionist, environmental engineer, equipment suppliers, university extension specialist, and so forth) and get a plan on paper of how a cattle mortality disaster will be handled on their operation. Their plan should include site selection; specific resources, including quantity of each (equipment, transportation, trenching needs, composting materials, and so forth); and availability of rendering. After the step-by-step plan is finished, it should be filed with the state's livestock control and environmental offices for review.

## CARCASS DISPOSAL METHODS

Seven methods of carcass disposal are discussed. These are packing plant slaughter, rendering, composting, burial, incineration, open burning, and hydrothermal carbonization. Only 4 of these methods currently have application after cattle mortalities have occurred (**Table 2**).

### Packing Plant Salvage Slaughter

There are 2 instances in which the packing plant salvage slaughter technique can be considered for cattle: a natural disaster (such as a tornado) that leaves large numbers of cattle injured or an emergency slaughter as part of an FAD control program managed by the USDA-APHIS-VS. Inquiries into emergency salvage slaughter as part of a USDA Food Safety Inspection Service–VS disease management plan should be made to the USDA-APHIS-VS.

Cattle considered for salvage slaughter after a disastrous storm must be transportable without inflicting additional injury or pain. As required by USDA Food Safety Inspection Service regulations, the cattle must be able to walk into a packing facility.

**Table 2**
**Disaster cattle disposal pros and cons**

| Disposal Method | Pros | Cons |
|---|---|---|
| Packing plant slaughter | Salvages some food value<br>Minimizes community concerns<br>Avoids all EPA disposal issues | Limited by packer availability and space<br>Must have both packer and USDA-FSIS approval, (USDA-APHIS-VS approval if a disease in involved) |
| Rendering | Salvages some meat by-product value<br>Minimizes community concerns<br>Avoids all EPA disposal issues | Limited by rendering availability |
| Composting | Can deal with a larger number of cattle than most other disposal techniques | Requires extensive resources (land and equipment)<br>Requires large carbon sources that may limited availability in cattle mortality disasters<br>EPA specifications must be met<br>Requires maintenance following disposal<br>The composting preprocess requires time (6 to 12 mo) |
| Burial | Can deal with a larger number of cattle than most other disposal techniques<br>The time required in relatively short compared to other disposal techniques | Requires significant resources (land and equipment)<br>EPA specifications must be met |
| Incineration pits | Can deal with a larger number of cattle than most other disposal techniques<br>The time required in relatively short compared to other disposal techniques | Significant EPA and community issues |
| Hydrothermal carbonization | Completely destroys all infectious disease pathogen DNA<br>Residual is easily disposed of without EPA concern | No units are currently available to handle large numbers of cattle mortalities |

There must not be any attempt to salvage slaughter downer cattle. To minimize pain and suffering of injured cattle, the decision should be made as soon as possible. Carcass trim loss in these situations can be substantial and have an impact on financial recovery from salvage slaughter. Cattle operations that have storm insurance for cattle loss need to contact their insurers to gain required permission for handling insured cattle and for getting needed documentation required for filing a claim.

*Rendering*

The availability of rendering services is variable across the United States, with the bulk available in livestock dense production areas. Rendering is an excellent way to recover some value from mortalities. Rendering does an excellent job of controlling pathogens and, with the exception of barbiturates, rendering temperatures denature all commonly used Food and Drug Administration–approved cattle medications, including sedatives, such as xylazine, and restraint medications, such as succinylcholine.[12–15]

Rendering, when available, is an excellent method of dealing with disaster mortalities. A potential limiting factor is the volume of mortalities that can overwhelm both transportation resources and rendering capacity. Blizzards followed by days or weeks of freezing temperatures provide an opportunity to stagger the delivery of carcasses to a rendering facility. Buying mortalities with additional snow helps preserve them. A stab incision through the abdominal wall before mortalities are buried with additional snow helps release gas and improve the stability of the carcass. As rendering space becomes available, carcasses can be uncovered and transported to rendering facilities.

The potential to use rendering after a natural disaster or in mortality emergencies should be included in an action plan. Important keys are not only the availability of rendering services but also transportation of mortalities to a rendering facility beyond the rendering trucks controlled by the rendering company. Cattle producer and farmer privately held flatbed trailers and trucks for hauling mortalities should be included in a disaster plan, but it is critical to get acknowledgment from these sources of their willingness to participate during a cattle mortality disaster.

### Burial

The practicality as well as feasibility of burying cattle carcass mortalities must be examined in the cattle mortality disposal plan. Burial plans must be carefully assessed by agriculture hydrologists and environmental agricultural engineers and then approved by the state's environmental protection agency. Carcass burial permit requirements vary and are subject to change; therefore, disaster planners must do assessment of permit requirements regularly. Fines for unauthorized cattle mortality burials could be substantial.

Principle among burial considerations is the potential for ground water contamination, which goes beyond just the depth of the water table. Soil structure; proximity to human dwellings, roads, and utilities, including water wells, pipelines, and electric lines; proximity to flood plains; and avoiding burial sites with greater than 5% slope are all critical factors in burial site selection.[16]

The number and depth of burial pits should be included in a cattle mortality disaster plan. Generally, pits are constructed to be the width of a bulldozer blade and approximately 8 ft to 10 ft deep.[16] Cattle mortality burial trenches require 6 ft of soil cover over the carcasses; therefore, a trench 10 ft deep provides 4 ft of depth for carcass disposal.[16] Each mature cattle carcass requires 2 cu yd to 3 cu yd of burial space, or 18 cu ft to 27 cu ft, and each linear foot of an 8-ft by 10-ft burial trench accommodates approximate 1.5 to 2 mature cattle carcasses. Therefore, 1000 cattle mortalities require 500 ft to 750 ft of linear trench space, with 80 cu ft of trench space per linear foot.

Although not critical, if possible all cattle carcasses should be vented prior to burial by making a stab or cut incision through the hide and piercing the abdomen. This allows decomposition gases to escape, thereby minimizing carcass swelling. This procedure aids in maintaining the integrity of the burial trench.

In addition to covering cattle carcasses with 6 ft of soil within the trench, it is advised to mound 2 ft to 3 ft of soil over the top of the burial trench. Diversion ditches should be constructed adjacent to carcass burial sites to prevent up slope water runoff from potentially entering the burial trench.[16] Burial trench locations must be recorded using Global Position Satellite coordinates and reported to the US

Emergency Response System. The trenched area should be fenced for at least a year to prevent animals or humans from accidental exposure to the burial site. Burial trenches must be regularly monitored for seepage. Over time, as the carcasses decompose, the trench surface retracts and additional soil will be needed to level the burial trench surface. Maintaining a mounded top over the burial trench aids in the protection of ground water.[16]

## Composting

Ongoing livestock mortality composting research provides a great deal of information regarding the utility of this disposal technique in animal agriculture settings. Fortunately, there have not been many large cattle mortality events in the United States to study. Although most available research only deals with a few mortalities, it does offer useful information to consider when planning for disposal of larger numbers of cattle mortalities in a disaster. As with all research, caution should be exercised when extrapolating research results to real-world application.

Composting should take place within the first 72 hours of loss of cattle life and is more complicated than some other carcass disposal methods. Therefore, advanced planning is required. The process is discussed briefly. More in-depth information can be found in the 2017 USDA-APHIS-VS Composting Livestock 2017: Livestock Mortality Composting Protocol.[17]

Composting basics include site selection, absorbent materials for a base, adequate organic material for the composting envelope (materials in immediate contact with the carcasses) to provide a carbon-to-nitrogen ratio greater than 25:1, and adequate moisture and material for a cap.

Carcass compost rows should be on higher ground but steep sloping terrain should be avoided. Maximum slope should be 2% to 4%. Sites that are relatively flat have advantages over steep sloping terrain.

The architecture of a mature cattle carcass compost pile is straightforward. **Fig. 7** demonstrates 3 different cattle composting technique designs for cattle: single layer; 3 cattle carcasses composted in triangle layering; and a 5-cattle carcass design. In all designs, it is important to have a base layer that is relatively dry, less than 40% moisture. The compost base should be approximately 18 in to 24 in thick. If the base material is dry, 18 in is sufficient, but 24 in may be needed if the base materials is slightly moist, such as semidry manure.[18]

Absorbent materials need to be available to build a base on which carcasses being composted will lay. Generally, materials with less than 35% moisture work. Common sources include ground corn stalks, straw, and/or dry manure. Although cattle operations may have what seems like a lot of manure and round bales, the quantity needed far exceeds the requirements demanded in a mortality disaster. To help planners prepare, the estimated composting requirements are provided in **Table 3**.

It is important in all designs for the envelope composting material used to surround the cattle carcasses to attain an approximate 8 in to 12 inches of separation between mature cattle carcasses. The separation distance can be reduced relative to the size of the cattle carcasses being composted. In the 5-cattle carcass design, a lined shallow trench serves to hold the compost pile base and as a cradle for the lowest layer of cattle carcasses. The material is distributed over the first carcasses to provide approximately 12 in of separation for the next mature cattle carcasses added to the pile. The separation distance can be reduced relative to the size of the cattle.

The organic material used for the envelope should be approximately 60% moisture. This moisture level feels wet but not so wet as to squeeze fluid from the material.[18] More than sufficient nitrogen is supplied by the decomposing carcasses.

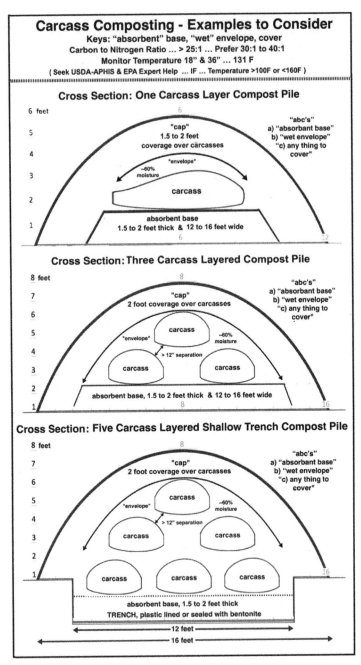

**Fig. 7.** Carcass compost design options.

Although there are many sources of carbon that can be used in carcass composting, such as plant and tree waste (mulch, ground stalks, and so forth), the most available source of carbon may be slightly moist manure (approximately 30%–40% moisture). Large cattle mortality disasters in which emergency composting might be

**Table 3**
**Carcass composting requirements (land and materials)**

| Number of Carcasses to Compost | Approximate Acres Needed (Including 200-ft Setback Perimeter Fence) | Absorbent Base Material Needed, Such as Round Bales (120 cu ft/ Round Bale) | Wet (Approximately 60% Moisture) Envelope Material Needed (cu yd) | Envelope Semidump Trailer Loads | Compost Row Cover (cu yd) | Cover Semidump Trailer Loads |
|---|---|---|---|---|---|---|
| 20 | 1/3 | 4–5 | 35–60 | 0.3–0.5 | 30 | 0.3–0.5 |
| 50 | 1/2 | 10–12 | 90–150 | 0.7–1 | 65 | .05–1 |
| 100 | 3/4 | 20–25 | 180–300 | 1.3–2.0 | 135 | 1–1.5 |
| 200 | 1 1/2 | 40–50 | 360–600 | 2.5–4.0 | 270 | 2–2.5 |
| 500 | 3 2/3 | 100–125 | 900–1500 | 6.3–10.5 | 670 | 5–6 |
| 750 | 5 1/4 | 150–170 | 1350–2250 | 9.5–16 | 1000 | 7–8 |
| 1000 | 7 | 200–250 | 1800–3000 | 13–21 | 1300 | 9–10 |
| 1500 | 11 1/2 | 300–375 | 2700–4500 | 19–32 | 2000 | 14–15 |
| 2000 | 15 | 400–500 | 3600–6000 | 25–42 | 2600 | 18–20 |
| 3000 | 20 1/4 | 600–750 | 5400–9000 | 38–63 | 3900 | 28–30 |
| 5000 | 35 | 1000–1250 | 9000–15,000 | 63–105 | 6700 | 45–50 |
| 10,000 | 70 | 2000–2500 | 18,000–30,000 | 125–210 | 13,000 | 90–100 |

Calculations from the author, D. Griffin. Disaster Cattle Composting Requirement Calculations Excel Spreadsheet, November 2017.
*Data from* USDA Composting Livestock 2017: livestock mortality composting protocol. USDA-APHIS, 2017.

considered and planned for most likely occur in areas with large numbers of cattle densely populated. Because the carbon-to-nitrogen ratio in slightly moist manure is lower than in plant material, more manure is required to cover composting carcasses and to absorb the leachate volume produced during decomposition of composted carcasses. If the carbon-to-nitrogen ratio is insufficient, less than 20:1, excessive nitrogen escapes the compost pile, resulting in objectionable odor emitted from the pile.[16,18]

If there is minimal disease transmission concern, all cattle carcasses should be vented prior to composting by making a stab or cut incision through the hide and piercing the abdomen. Venting allows decomposition gases to escape, which minimizes carcass swelling and aids with maintaining the integrity of the composting pile (**Box 2**).[18]

To help protect the composting carcasses, a cap or cover, known as the biofilter layer should be built over the row after the last carcasses have been added and covered with moist envelope material. The cap or cover should typically be 18 in to 24 in thick. It is best if the biofilter is organic material, such as dry to moist manure, but dirt is acceptable.

It is critical to maintain an adequate cover (biofilter) over the compost pile and to monitor the internal compost pile temperature using a thermometer with a 3-ft to 4-ft stem. The average temperature 18 in to 36 in within the compost pile should reach at least 131°F for at least 72 hours. If the internal temperature falls below 100°F or exceeds 160°F for 72 hours, a USDA-APHIS-VS and state environmental protection agency approved composting expert (subject matter expert) should be contacted to assess possible corrective measures.[18]

> **Box 2**
> **Composting material needs thumb rules**
>
> - Per 1,000 lb, approximately 6 cu yd with 35:40 carbon-to-nitrogen ratio
> - Per 1,000 lb, approximately 9 cu yd to 12 cu yd if the carbon-to-nitrogen ratio is less than 30:1
>   - 9000 yd to 12,000 yd per 1000 adult cattle mortalities
>   - If using slightly moist manure, the higher yardage value is required.
> - Typical semidump trailers haul 35 yd to 45 yd.
> - 250 to 300 semidump trailers per 1000 adult cattle mortalities
> - Per 1,000 lb, requires 2.5 to 3.5 linear feed, 12-ft to 16-ft wide compost row
> - 12 ft to 16 ft needed between compost rows
> - 1000 adult cattle mortalities require 10, 300-ft rows
> - Compost areas require a 200-ft protection perimeter.
> - 10 acres needed per 1000 adult cattle mortalities

Objectionable odor is an indication that gaseous nitrogen is leaking from the compost pile and is likely associated with a carbon-to-nitrogen ratio less than 20:1. If objectionable odor is detected, additional organic matter should be applied to the composting pile.[18]

### Incineration and Open Burning

Carcass incineration units are not designed to handle the volume of cattle mortalities after a natural disaster. Open burning of cattle mortalities after a natural disaster is not permissible without permitting by state and federal environmental agencies. Additionally, it is important to remember, less than 1% of the US population is directly involved in animal agriculture and, therefore, the social and political pushback from open carcass burning could be enormous. If open carcass burning is considered in the state and/or county emergency carcass disposal plan, federal, state, and local regulations must be regularly evaluated. Fuel requirements should be assessed relative to current area cattle populations and funding sources secured. Burning 1 cattle carcass requires approximately 1 gallon of fuel oil.[16] The National Animal Health Management System guidelines (USDA, 2005)[19] have an extensive section on carcass burning considerations. Environmentally, burning may be a better choice than burial if ground water tables are high and ground water contamination is a potential concern. Burning mortality carcasses may also be a reasonable consideration if rendering services are not available and composting is not possible.[16]

### Hydrothermal Carbonization

The recent development of hydrothermal carbonization may in the future play a role in disposal of cattle mortalities after a disaster.[19] The concept includes having several hydrothermal carbonization reactors strategically located in the United States that could be deployed to a disaster area to deal with livestock mortalities on-site. Once reactors are in place at the disaster location, they can be operational within 24 hours to 36 hours. The reactors should be able to effectively not only deal with large volumes of cattle mortalities but also destroy all animal disease pathogens and animal DNA. The byproduct of the reactors is fluid that can be stored and transported to another location for additional processing.[17]

## DEALING WITH MORTALITIES AND EUTHANASIA

Both euthanasia and disposal of mass animal numbers generate serious emotional wellness issues. This should be factored in preparedness, response, and recovery. For more information, see Erin Wasson and Audry Wieman's article "Mental Health During Environmental Crises and Mass Fatality Events," in this issue.

## SUMMARY

The 2013 AVMA guidelines list the following as acceptable methods of euthanasia in cattle: (1) overdose of a barbiturate, (2) gunshot, and (3) penetrating or nonpenetrating CB (for calves and young animals only), with adjunctive methods to assure death. Multiple drawbacks to euthanasia by barbiturate overdose encourage consideration of the physical methods of gunshot and CB. People who may be required to euthanize an animal must know the proper anatomic site for conducting the procedure, be able to accurately interpret the physical indicators of unconsciousness and apply adjunctive methods to assure death, and, last but not least, be able to confirm death. Finally, over the years, either from ignorance or out of convenience, people have resorted to the use of methods deemed unacceptable for euthanasia. Veterinarians have a professional as well as moral obligation to correct such practices and insure a humane death for animals.

Beyond the importance of ensuring a humane death for animals in disaster situations is safeguarding the environment and human health and safety through the proper disposal of animal carcasses. Carcass disposal options include packing plant slaughter, rendering, composting, burial, incineration, open burning, and hydrothermal carbonization. Open pyre burning requires special permitting, and incineration is likely too costly for mass casualties. Although still being developed, hydrothermal carbonization is a method that may be useful in the future for dealing with cattle mortalities after disaster situations.

## REFERENCES

1. American Veterinary Medical Association. AVMA guidelines on Euthanasia, 2013 edition. Available at: https://www.avma.org/KB/Policies/Documents/euthanasia. pdf. Accessed April 6, 2018.
2. Fulwider WK, Grandin T, Rollin BE, et al. Survey of management practices on one hundred and thirteen north central and northeastern United States dairies. J Dairy Sci 2008;91:1686–92.
3. Humane Slaughter Association. Humane killing of livestock using firearms, guidance notes #3. 2nd edition. Wheathampstead (United Kingdom): Humane Slaughter Association; 1999.
4. Baker HJ, Scrimgeour HJ. Evaluation of methods for the euthanasia of cattle in a foreign animal disease outbreak. Can Vet J 1995;36:160–5.
5. Thomson DU, Wileman BW, Rezac DJ, et al. Computed tomographic evaluation to determineefficacy of euthanasia of yearling feedlot cattle by use of various firearm-ammunition combinations. Am J Vet Res 2013;74(11):1385–91.
6. Gilliam JN, Woods J, Hill J, et al. Evaluation of the cash euthanizer captive bolt system as a single step euthanasia method for cattle of various ages. 4th International Symposium on Beef Cattle Welfare. Ames, IA, July 16-18, 2014.
7. AVMA guidelines for the humane slaughter of animals: 2016 edition. Available at: https://www.avma.org/KB/Resources/Reference/AnimalWelfare/Documents/ Humane-Slaughter-Guidelines.pdf. Accessed April 6, 2018.

8. Gilliam JN, Shearer JK, Woods J, et al. Captive-bolt euthanasia of cattle: determination of optimal-shot placement and evaluation of the cash special euthanizer kit® for euthanasia of cattle. Anim Welfare 2012;21(S2):99–102.

9. Dewell RD, Bear DA, Weber W, et al. Description and justification of a consistent technique for euthanasia of bovines using firearm and penetrating captive bolt. Bovine Pract 2016;50(2):190–5.

10. Finnie JW, Manavis J, Blumbergs PC, et al. Brain damage in sheep from penetrating captive bolt stunning. Aust Vet J 2002;80(1 & 2):67–9.

11. Evers AS, Crowder CM, Balser JR. General anesthetics. In: Brunton LL, Lazo JS, Parker KL, editors. Goodman and Gillman's the pharmacological basis of therapeutics. 11th edition. New York: McGraw-Hill Medical Publishing Division; 2006. p. 362.

12. Miller LP, Moore KJ, Lemieux PM. Foreign animal disease preparedness & response plan, standard operational procedures 14. Disposal. Dearborn (MI): USDA-APHIS-VS; 2014.

13. Bērziņs A, Krūkle K, Actiņs A, et al. The relative stability of xylazine hydrochloride polymorphous forms. Pharm Dev Technol 2010;15(2):217–22.

14. Chiu L, Parasrampuria J, Bommireddi A, et al. Moist-heat sterilization and the chemical stability of heat-labile parenteral solutions. Drug Dev Ind Pharm 1998; 24(1):89–93.

15. Fanco DA. Animal disposal: the environmental, animal disease, and public health related implications: an assessment of options, California Dept. of Food Agriculture. Symposium, Sacramento, CA, April 8, 2002.

16. Ducey TF, Collins KS, Woodbury BL, et al. Hydrothermal carbonization of livestock mortality for the reduction of pathogens and microbially-derived DNA. Front Environ Sci Eng 2017;11(3):9.

17. Miller LP, Buckendahl A, Flory GA, et al. USDA composting technical committee: composting livestock 2017: livestock mortality composting protocol. Riverdale (MD): USDA-APHIS; 2017.

18. Woodbury BL. Large-scale disposal of animal mortalities. Clay Center (NB): US-Meat Anim Res Cent Meet Notes; 2017.

19. APHIS Veterinary Services (VS) Writing Group. National animal health emergency management system guidelines, operational guidelines. Disposal, USDA. Riverdale (MD): USDA-APHIS-VS; 2005.

# Mental Health During Environmental Crisis and Mass Incident Disasters

Erin Wasson, BSW, MSW, RSW[a],*, Audry Wieman, DVM[b]

## KEYWORDS

- Agriculture • Disaster • Mental health • Emergency • Veterinarian • Client • Support

## KEY POINTS

- Preparation for the mental stresses of veterinary medicine combined with increased education in mental health may be protective factors for veterinarians in times of disaster.
- Veterinarians are first responders in times of environmental or mass incident disaster in the treatment of animals.
- Mental health concerns are common during catastrophic events and may develop immediately or take weeks or months to manifest.
- As trusted members of agricultural communities, veterinarians are sought for psychosocial support and should equip themselves with referral information for clients in cases where mental health is impacted during disaster response.
- Learning how to approach clients and colleagues about mental health and familiarizing oneself with rural and remote support services is key to client safety and service provision.

## INTRODUCTION

Veterinary medicine has a unique role in times of crisis when environmental factors or mass incident disasters lead to herd injury or death. Events that cause large-scale livestock deaths include natural disasters and depopulation because of infectious disease. Livestock veterinarians are immersed in their communities during disasters and are subjected to unique experiences, effects, and challenges. Although the primary role of the livestock veterinarian is to manage the health and welfare of the animals, secondary roles have emerged and are documented in the literature. Distressed clients expect veterinarians provide medical expertise and social support during decision-making processes related to animal health.[1,2] As a result,

---

The authors have nothing to disclose.
[a] Veterinary Social Work Program, Western College of Veterinary Medicine, University of Saskatchewan, 52 Campus Drive, Saskatoon, SK S7N5B4, Canada; [b] Ridgeline Vet Services, LLC, 89493 509th Avenue, Lynch, NB 68746, USA
* Corresponding author.
*E-mail address:* erin.wasson@usask.ca

veterinarians often end up managing the distress of their clients, and their own reactions to mass incident and environmental crises and that of their family and colleagues. Veterinarians and paraprofessionals have recently begun to partner their expertise to bridge those clients struggling with mental health concerns to appropriate professional assessment and support.

## AWARENESS AND IMPORTANCE OF MENTAL HEALTH

*When I got there they were all dead. All of them. We didn't have a good answer for them yet. We couldn't figure out why. We just knew that today we would be focused on burying them and disposing of their bodies. We'd have to wait to see what the tests showed. What it was that killed them. Everyone was really angry and really sad*

—*Veterinary team member reflecting on mass incident*

### Veterinarians as First Responders

Because of the presence of animals in most geographic locations, veterinarians are often among the first responders during environmental disasters.[3] Livestock veterinarians and their staff shoulder long hours, intense interactions with frightened and injured livestock, high volumes of euthanasia, communications with distraught clients, and the implications of the disaster on the future of their own business and the businesses of their clients. First responder groups are known to be at a higher risk of experiencing acute stress disorder (ASD) reactions because of distressing events and post-traumatic stress disorder (PTSD) resulting from accumulated experiences or occurrences of trauma witnessed as a part their duties.[4–6] Veterinarians are often closely intertwined with the owners of the animals and the community where the event occurs. This intimacy can intensify the impact of dealing with such stressful incidences. Veterinarians are likely to minimize the emotional impact on themselves and "dedicate themselves to work, sacrifice rest and respite, and risk exhaustion and burn-out."[7] Although veterinary medical assistance teams have been deployed during devastating disasters, such as 9/11 and the flooding in Texas caused by Tropical storm Allison, the emotional and psychological impacts on these emergency preparedness teams have not been evaluated.[3,8] Although each person may respond differently to these large-scale incidents, the impact is felt by all who experience it. As a result, it is warranted that veterinarians understand the existing stressors in rural communities during times of calm, to understand why an escalation in stress and trauma uniquely impacts on these communities.

### Farm Stress

Farm stress as a general concept has been well documented in the literature.[9–13] Writers cite financial pressure, poor psychological work environments, vulnerability to changes in weather, interest rates, debt load, and competing work and home responsibilities as contributing to the stressors experienced.[9–14] The reported results of these stressors include increased levels of anxiety, depression, poor coping generally, and in some cases suicide.[9,11–14] A 2005 study confirmed that nearly two-thirds farmers surveyed identified feelings of stress associated with farming. Moreover, "one in five farmers described themselves as being very stressed while almost half describe themselves as being somewhat stressed."[1]

The identified farm stress explored in the literature refers only to generalized feelings of stress associated with farming and not acute incidences. Because farmers identify at high risk for stress generally, it would follow that during times of mass incident or environmental disaster, this sector would experience greater vulnerability and increased risk for psychological injury. This is evident in the literature. A 2004 study of the impact of an outbreak ovine Johne disease in Australia, identified that farmers reported feelings of trauma, stigma, a sense of personal failure, loss of identity, diminished self-esteem, and family disruption as a result of the authoritarian administration of aid programs, and poorly handled testing programs, which caused feelings of confusion, stress, and anger.[15] The reported mental health outcomes included depression, PTSD, and suicide. One farmer was quoted as saying "I used to think of the killing fields. They were in Cambodia. I now know they are here. I can't go back into that paddock"[15]; and another as saying "My wife has been into the paddock three times with a car full of petrol and a hose and couldn't commit suicide...that is, what is going on."[15] Further damages experienced by the communities constituted multiple losses and included damage to economic, relational, community, and familial structures.[15] Similar experiences are reported in a Dutch dairy farm study, where as a result of foot and mouth disease approximately one-half of farmers experienced PTSD after their animals were culled.[16] In a survey of Australia's first equine influenza outbreak respondents described psychological distress at five times the level reported in local population health data.[17] Although the bond between human beings and companion animals is largely understood to be an interconnected part of human existence,[18-20] it is also more commonly accepted that the death of a companion animal is experienced similarly to the death of a human counterpart.[21-23] Within agriculture there is an increased likelihood of experiencing disenfranchised grief, where the relationship, the loss, or the griever goes unrecognized and where loss is not socially validated.[24,25] Decisions to cull may increase feelings of regret, guilt, or feelings of failure, particularly in disease control where otherwise healthy animals are culled as a means of managing an outbreak.[7] As a result, the self-stigma combined with beliefs around mental health may pose barriers to accessing support. For these reasons, it is pertinent that veterinarians be aware of the common stress responses associated with traumatic events that may impact on their clients.

### Mental Health Responses to Trauma

ASD and PTSD are two common mental health diagnoses after incidences of mass casualty.[26-28] These conditions can affect people that have no other mental health history, and stem from the individual's response to the trauma exposure.[28] Authors note that struggles associated with trauma-induced mental illnesses are thought to revolve around the concept of moral injury.[29] In the case of a traumatic event, the injury is incurred to an individual's belief system or moral code, whereby that person cannot mentally or emotionally resolve the dichotomy between their beliefs and the event that was witnessed.[29]

Practitioners state that ASD typically manifest in the first 4 weeks after the incident and may affect from 14% to 33% of the exposed population.[30] Typically, symptoms are psychological and physical in nature. The psychological features include[30]

- Horror
- Dissociative symptoms (detachment, depersonalization, dissociative amnesia, and decreased awareness)
- Re-experiencing the event
- Depression
- Avoidance behaviors

Physical symptoms may include[30]

- Fatigue
- Insomnia
- Headaches
- Gastrointestinal (upset stomach)
- Cardiovascular (hypertension, stroke, cardiac arrest)
- Rheumatic conditions (inflammatory issues)

Although ASD may predispose some individuals to PTSD, it is not always a precursor to PTSD. PTSD develops at least 4 weeks after the trauma but may not present for months or even years after the event.[26,31,32] Similar to some physical injuries, mental injuries may take longer to surface. PTSD shares many symptoms with ASD, and some of the same treatments. However, authors suggest that a major difference, beyond onset, is that there is less exhibition of dissociative symptoms and more prevalence of anxiety, depression, and physical disturbances.[31] Other mental health issues may also occur during or after catastrophic events including major depressive disorder, anxiety, survivor's guilt, and alcohol and substance misuse. Some additional signs include[29]

- Emotional swings including angry outburst and loss of patience
- Insomnia
- Excessively increasing or decreasing workloads
- Reduced social contact or isolation
- General distress
- Relationship or parenting issues
- Loss of spirituality or faith; reckless, violent behavior

It is not uncommon for trauma responses to be delayed after exposure. These symptoms may not present until after the clean-up efforts have begun or been completed and the chronicity of the event begins to weigh on those affected. For this reason, exposed individuals should be periodically evaluated for changes in their emotional state. In some cases, instinctual avoidance behaviors and strategies tend to alleviate stress in the immediate period following trauma.[29] If an individual persists in avoiding processing a traumatic event, then issues can develop into more destructive outcomes long term.[29,33] Early recognition of clinical signs is important in aiding people with ASD and PTSD to recover.[29] Veterinarians and their support staff should be aware of risk to their own, colleague, and producer mental health during and after events.[32]

To build resilience, practitioners must be able to communicate well with clients and others associated with the intervention. Debriefing smaller scale incidences can further prepare veterinarians and their teams for positive outcomes. Open conversations increase resiliency to stress and normalize the process in the case of a massive event. Historically the veterinary profession has not invested in communication training for students. The literature notes that veterinarians as a profession have limited preparation or training in the area of communication to aid in supporting and managing the social aspects of veterinary practice.[34] Feeling a lack of ability, knowledge, or uncertainty about how to appropriately direct clients in distress is a source of significant stress for veterinarians. Training related to communication is changing and some universities are implementing simulated client interactions and advanced communication education.[35] This measure responds to the social side of veterinary medicine teaching skills that bridge their clients with appropriate mental health resources.[36] The ability to create this connection relieves the pressure on veterinarians of working beyond their scope of expertise and create a positive relationship with clients by removing barriers to access of qualified support services.[36]

## STRATEGIES AND INTERVENTIONS
### Interventions for Community Members and Clients

*How do I introduce you? What do I say?*
*—Veterinarian to mental health provider*

A range of interventions are available to manage farm stress including education and more traditional counseling support.[10–12] It is not uncommon that individuals in the community that are seen as reliable, resilient, problem-solvers, and good listeners are sought for comfort. Friends, family, medical professionals, and clergy that display these characteristics become the primary sources of comfort and healing in rural communities. In times where there is widespread disaster, such as floods, tornadoes, and fires, these more informal resources become strained as confidantes are simultaneously managing their own exposure to events. Some individuals may be naturally resilient, cope well, and be able to manage on their own. Still others may need professional support. Although assessment and treatment are best left to professional counselors, colleagues and friends can provide valuable empathy and redirect those members of the community who are more heavily affected to appropriate services.[33]

Veterinarians should avoid mental health diagnosis or determining if an individual needs professional help. Instead, veterinarians should focus on reducing stigma, normalizing access to services, and enhancing their own knowledge of local service providers. There are certain characteristics of those who provide support that allow for maximum healing. Critical to the ability to provide support is sensitivity and understanding of the unique cultural characteristics of these communities, particularly for those veterinarians who come from urban settings.[2,7] In particular this means valuing[37]

- The self-sufficiency of families
- Traditional gender roles
- The presence and value of multigenerational families
- Children as active working participants
- Attachment to the legacy of the farm
- Strong work ethics
- A connection to land and animals
- Reluctance or resistance to change
- A stoic presentation

As a result, these families are often more highly resourced and may be less likely to seek outside support particularly in areas where mental health practitioners may be more challenging to access because of geographic, temporal, or transportation barriers.[7]

In times of distress, it benefits veterinarians to provide their clients with redirection to those support services known to understand and connect well to rural culture. Although sometimes beyond the comfort of the veterinary/client relationship boundaries, clients share their reactions to traumatic circumstances. Clients that repeatedly tell their experiences are attempting to accommodate their feelings and process the event.[38] Restraint from nonverbal and verbal judgements about an individual's experience, actions, or feelings about an experience is key. Veterinarians can provide these people with a list of local professional support systems and protect themselves, simultaneously, by relieving the pressure of managing client mental health.[33]

During a major disaster, psychological first aid is a series of steps that aims to provide a way to ensure safety for individuals experiencing symptoms of ASD. The goal is to provide practical assistance from first responders at the time of severe trauma and help normalize the individual's responses to trauma. Psychological first aid recommends that to appropriately support someone in a time a trauma one should[33]

- Contact the individual and engage warmly
- Establish that the individual is safe
- Calm and orient the individual
- Gather information on needs and concerns nonjudgmentally
- Provide practical assistance to address those needs and concerns
- Connect with social support systems (friends and family)
- Provide coping information if possible
- Link the individual with collaborative services (eg, recovery assistance, public sector services, mental health organizations, medical access)

Assuming that the trauma survivor will seek professional support creates barriers in rural communities where there is significant stigma around mental health. The independent nature of farmers and the lack of experienced rural health providers also serve as barriers.[12] Veterinarians are in regular contact with these producers and are professionals with whom the client feels comfortable discussing medical topics. Studies show that farmers who are interested in receiving support are nearly doubly more likely to access services from a professional known to them than a sibling, spouse, friend, or stress counselor.[39] A connection with local mental health systems should be established to compile a list of low-cost, mobile, 24-hour and distance services that provide immediate opportunities for support. Curating a list of available supports in the communities in which veterinarians work, before a time of crisis, is imperative to this planning. This readiness may provide the window to a client's openness that encourages them to take a step toward professional help. Normalizing the individual's reaction to a distressing event and simultaneously redirecting them reduces the stigma and empowers the producer to determine their need for themselves. For some veterinarians, these conversations may become awkward. Preparing for these interactions may ease some of the discomfort and allow the veterinarian to give relevant information to a concerned producer. **Box 1** provides a guide to begin the practice of having these conversations.[40]

These writers recommend that should a veterinarian wish to expand on their ability to appropriately redirect clients, that they invest in accessing further continuing

---

**Box 1**
**Opening statements for veterinarians offering support**

*Connect* "This situation has been just (awful, horrible, shocking, terrifying)"

*Empathize* "It makes sense you're feeling the way you are, given everything that has happened"

*Elicit* "What changes have you noticed about yourself since this has happened?"

*Reflect* "Sounds like you're not sure how to manage all of this"

*Normalize* "Seems to me that just about anybody who's had to go through this might need a hand"

*Offer* "How about I leave you a list of people you could contact if you needed someone to talk to, just in case you ever wanted it?"

education in psychological first aid or mental health first aid, as a means of increasing skill and comfort in providing intermediary support in times of crisis.[33]

### National Programs and Services

National programs and services can provide a valuable resource to those veterinarians working in isolated areas. Within the United States, the US Department of Health and Human Services offers information and support for those experiencing a mental health concern at www.mentalhealth.gov.[41] All US citizens can access service providers through the SAMHSA treatment referral helpline (1-877-SAMHSA7).[42] Also the national suicide prevention hotline is available for immediate intervention (1-800-273-TALK or www.suicidepreventionlifeline.org). If an individual is at imminent risk for suicide ensure the person is taken to the nearest emergency room.

Within Canada crisis centers vary province by province. Fortunately the LifeLine foundation has compiled a list of resources (link in references).[43] In addition, the provinces of Saskatchewan, Manitoba, and Prince Edward Island have available farm stress hotlines that can provide immediate assistance in times of distress.[39] Quality mental health services are available country-wide and are accessed through 211 (www.211.ca), a primary source for accessing information on all government, community-based, and social services.[44] Both in Canada and the United States, larger organizations, such as the red cross (www.redcross.org), provide access to services in affected areas.[45] Veterinarians can benefit from researching the services provided by disaster relief organizations to better equip themselves with resource information.

### Interventions for Veterinarians

It is well known that the veterinary profession has struggled with high incidences of mental health–related concerns.[46–49] Veterinarians put the welfare of others before their own and this has significant short- and long-term repercussions. Additional risk factors for veterinary mental health disruption include a drive for high-performance and perfectionist qualities.[47] They also face irregular working hours, overwhelming workloads, high expectations and demands from clients, and working in psychologically and physically isolating environments.[46] Emergency preparedness teams are often rapidly created for emergency veterinary work, but preparing them for the mental rigors and debriefing them after the incident is an area that is still under development. It is pertinent that veterinarians consider how their practice and personal lives (friends and family) are impacted when they are processing the aftermath of a disaster. External support should be sought by the veterinarian or their staff if they are struggling. Recovery from these mental injuries is necessary to promote personal well-being, career longevity, and ethical professional practice. Next are some strategies developed as a mechanism to prepare veterinarians and other team members for crisis response interventions with livestock to limit and prevent damage caused by traumatic exposure (**Box 2**).[50]

### Boundaries and Threshold for Managing Crisis

During times of crisis, it is not uncommon for responders to reach a point where they can no longer safely intervene. Veterinarians should consider their threshold for managing the stressors of a traumatic event and determine whether they can continue to provide services safely. As a crisis unfolds, it is challenging to see the larger picture. Responders may struggle to identify that they have reached overexposure to crisis and can no longer work effectively. Veterinarians must understand key features of empathy fatigue and watch for these within themselves as a measure of safety. Awareness of these reactions alerts responders to the need to stop work. The American

**Box 2**
**Preparation for exposure**

*Before*

- *Enhance team skills* through the completion of psychological first aid or by adding paraprofessionals (eg, social workers, psychologists) to the team.

- *Participants should determine whether they should be involved.* Some people are comfortable providing services and some are not (multiple euthanasia, information on body disposal). There are some things you cannot "unsee" or you may have reached your threshold for cases you can attend to; know your limit and practice within it.

- *Get clear on what feels worrisome* in anticipation of the event; discuss as a team how you intend to manage these issues if they come up. This helps the team assign tasks, be aware of each other's triggers, and lays groundwork for supporting one another.

- *Discuss goals* of interventions (eg, manage disease, mitigate welfare concerns).

- *Discuss how the day will go* in detail. Include leadership roles, tasks, duties, methods, rotating through tasks to avoid overexposure, tasks team members cannot do (physically, emotionally, or otherwise), break times, any other ideas that emerge from earlier discussion.

- *Plan activities for the days end.* These should be activities that members of the team find restore a sense of hope. Some examples include spending time with children or pets, time spent in nature away from disaster, time spent in solitude and reflection, and spiritual practices. These should be activities that are an individual fit for participants and should be decided on by each member before attending. Team leaders should check-in, throughout the period of exposure, to ensure team members are active in their self-care.

*During*

- *Start with self-care* each day, ensuring that team members are engaging in the necessary activities to promote good mental health.

- *Good organization is key.* Implement the plans organized during the before stage. Diligence in cataloging, processing, and treating animals is important. Creating flow in the work so that it can go as smoothly as possible is imperative (when the processes are smooth it can allow participants to appropriately disconnect so that they may cope effectively with tasks). Ensuring clear methodology during the process should remove some decision-making pressure from participants. Ensure participants are in roles that they can manage and that participants are relieved of/changing roles throughout the day.

- *Take a break.* Throughout the day this will seem challenging. It is imperative that breaks are taken to look after participants, change processes that are not working well, allow for team member role changes, and to gain some distance from tasks at hand.

- *Coordinate with other first responders* to lessen the impact on the veterinary team through reduced professional isolation.

- *At the end of each day* the team should meet to reflect on what went well and what did not, implementing change where current processes inhibit work flow.

*After*

- *Debrief.* Someone in a leadership role needs to lead this discussion. Discuss first what was challenging, then what the team believed went well. Discussing challenges and then discussing how you coped with them is important. When discussing what went well, the focus is not about "putting a shine on it," but instead focusing on the necessity of the work (eg, relieving distress or preventing potential disease/spread of disease). Consider hiring outside support to facilitate this portion if leadership is not clear, there has been team conflict, or team leaders are depleted and cannot perform this task.

- *Offer/Access professional support.* As with clients, the participants need to also feel as though they are able to access support for themselves if need be. Compile a list of local resources to provide team members. Encourage team members to access this support regardless of each member's perception of their ability to manage.

Veterinary Medical Association describes compassion fatigue as having the following qualities[51]:

- Bottled-up emotions
- Sadness and apathy
- Inability to get pleasure from activities that previously were enjoyable
- Isolation
- Difficulty concentrating
- Feeling mentally and physically tired
- Chronic physical ailments; voicing excessive complaints about your job, your manager, and/or coworkers
- Lack of self-care, including poor hygiene and a drop-off in your appearance
- Recurring nightmares or flashbacks
- Substance abuse or other compulsive behaviors, such as overeating or gambling

The veterinary literature neglects professional boundaries as they pertain to setting limits during times of disaster. When under prolonged pressure, effectiveness is reduced. Practitioners experiencing the symptoms of empathy fatigue during a traumatic event have reached their threshold for service provision. Veterinarians who recognize an increase in empathy fatigue or mental health injury must invest in their own resilience before providing further care to others.[33] This may mean that despite there being no end in sight to the crisis, veterinarians may have to reduce involvement. Additionally, this may mean that veterinarians explore other team-based options with surrounding veterinary clinics rotating involvement to ensure that each provider has time away from the crisis to provide general wellness services (spend time with generally healthy animals) or rest. Negative reactions to the work environment represent a creeping violation to the practitioner's boundaries. Burnout is identified by the emotional exhaustion, depersonalization, and reduced sense of accomplishment felt by a service provider.[52] Literature on burnout suggests people pursue equity and reciprocity in their relationships and there is an assumption that there is a personal gain in return for investment in work.[53] Authors suggest that the feelings of equity are at-risk when investments, whether they be of time, skill, effort, or attention, exceed gains.[53] In times of crisis investment exceeds gain in the short term, and responders are at risk of feelings of inequity associated with burnout. This is particularly apparent in crisis situations where elevated needs meet scarce resources and where a strained relationship between sociopolitical spheres leads to moral distress.[54]

Much emphasis has been placed on the need to engage in self-care as a part of veterinary practice.[55,56] Self-care is by definition the activities undertaken by the individuals, families, and communities, on their own or in partnership with professional supports, to enhance health, prevent disease, limit illness, and restore health.[57] Engaging in self-care is challenging when it is not a priority or where mental health injury has already occurred. As a result, it is recommended that if confronted with these challenges, veterinarians seek professional support to aid in self-care planning.

## DISCUSSION
### Barriers and Considerations

Few programs are available specifically for veterinarians and staff that address trauma responses and other mental health issues following catastrophic events. Some state/provincial veterinary medical associations provide visible access to mental health care, whereas other states are lacking in accessible information.[58] One barrier to rural mental health care for livestock veterinarians is the lack of competent service providers. Many counselors do not understand rural culture and have difficulty making connections to the people they are trying to help. Conversely, some practitioners are so well known within the community that they fear accessing support because of concerns of confidentiality and stigma. These concerns are similar to rural community members who fear judgment for accessing services and are wary of practitioner's ability to provide confidential support. Although mental health has been a historically taboo subject, its existence in every population is undeniable. Providing a case for definition, diagnosis, treatment, and prevention options is the same as with other medical issues. Large-scale disasters are the prime events for outside services to provide necessary and effective care for the individuals impacted by the disaster. It is for this reason that veterinarians should enhance their understanding of mental health and learn to collaborate with paraprofessionals.

There is need to address the fact that many rural communities go underserved in terms of access to mental health support. Authors note that rural communities consistently have higher unmet mental health needs than their urban counterparts.[59] Studies have shown that there are challenges in retaining mental health practitioners in rural areas leading to increased impediments in service provision.[60] During times of mass incident or environmental crisis the need to provide geographically sensitive and immediate support is a necessity. Many mental health practitioners work from a fixed office space. This can pose a barrier to service provision in time of mass incident or environmental disaster. Often community members who are managing clean up–associated herd culls and disposal of livestock are unable to commute to distant services. When asked, producers remark that until mental health providers attend and directly, "get boots on the ground," and see what they are coping with, they do not feel truly understood. For these reasons it is of benefit for mental health providers to consider how community outreach could help increase access and rapport to appropriately service rural and remote communities. Some examples include public service agencies attending fundraising events associated with disasters; mobile teams attending to disaster sites; and mental health providers seeking access to these communities through trusted service providers, such as veterinarians.

## SUMMARY: FUTURE RESEARCH AND OPPORTUNITIES IN CURRICULUM

Beyond direct practice, there are gaps in mental health education. Core concepts of community-based practice, crisis intervention, rural and remote cultural norms, and the issues that arise in the connections between human beings and animals are integral to preparing students to manage environmental crisis and mass incident. It is therefore important that those institutions responsible for educating future generations of mental health providers consider the implications of including rural content. Within veterinary medicine, further education and research should focus on enhancing resiliency and providing tactics to prevent traumatic injury. At minimum education related to managing professional boundaries to support good mental health should be considered.

Building resiliency to adverse events has become an increasingly important part the curriculum in medical professions.[38] Developing better personal coping mechanisms is extremely beneficial to graduates once they are out of school and in a more isolated environment. Studies focused on attributes of individuals that manage stress well have identified several factors that explain resilience.[38] Self-efficacy, composure, and planning allow an individual to manage setbacks without excessive anxiety.[38] These skills are developed during times of lower stress and allow people to effectively prepare for more stressful events. Self-efficacy is encouraged through allowing a veterinarian the opportunity to attempt and complete new goals. Planning for emergencies gives individuals a foundational knowledge of what to expect and effective responses to scenarios. Composure may be developed through recognizing stressors and implementing relaxation techniques.[38] Perseverance through smaller stressful events contributes to the belief that an individual can have a positive impact on an overwhelming event.[38]

Some work has been done to offer preventative education and coping mechanisms to prepare veterinary students for the trials they may face in practice. The University of Tennessee developed a suicide prevention Web site and collaborated with their College of Social Work to develop programs to help veterinarians prepare for the rigors of the profession.[61] Through their Suicide Awareness in Veterinary Education (S. A. V. E.) program, students learn curriculum in classrooms and through self-study online as a means of increasing mental health education.[61] Zoetis has also added new modules related to personal wellness in the catalog of courses offered through VETVANCE to support good mental health.[62] Inclusion of core mental health curriculum within accredited veterinary programs, as a preventative measure, is one method of addressing these concerns. There is an opportunity to better equip veterinary students through curriculum expansion that addresses inadequacy related to disaster relief and disaster response. Veterinarians in the field should be equipped to respond to mass incidents and disasters, and the everyday psychological burdens of the profession. It is well understood that preventative medicine is an important tenant of medicine. Preparing the veterinary community for mental health wellness and partnership with paraprofessionals is an opportunity that should be not be overlooked.

## REFERENCES

1. Western Opinion Research. National stress and mental survey of Canadian farmers: report to the Canadian Agricultural Safety Association. 2005. Available at: http://www.ruralsupport.ca/admin/FileUpload/files/publications/NationalStressSurvey ResultsPublic2005.pdf?PHPSESSID=d6b6b106528c8e703ff173aa1aa04d79. Accessed August 30, 2017.

2. Morrissey SA, Reser JP. Natural disasters, climate change and mental health considerations for rural Australia. Aust J Rural Health 2007;15(2):120–5.

3. Nolen S. VMATs aid rescue efforts in New York City. American Veterinary Medical Association. 2001. Available at: www.avma.org/onlnews/%0Ajavma/nov01/s110101a.asp%0A%0A. Accessed October 11, 2017.

4. Shepherd D, McBride D, Lovelock K. First responder well-being following the 2011 Canterbury earthquake. Disaster Prev Manag An Int J 2017;26(3):286–97.

5. Perrin MA, DiGande L, Wheeler K, et al. Differences in PTSD prevalence and associated risk factors among World Trade Center disaster rescue and recovery workers. Am J Psychiatry 2007;164(9):1385–94.

6. Boffa JW, Stanley IH, Hom MA, et al. PTSD symptoms and suicidal thoughts and behaviors among firefighters. J Psychiatr Res 2017;84:277–83.

7. Hall MJ, Ng A, Ursano RJ, et al. Psychological impact of the animal-human bond in disaster preparedness and response. J Psychiatr Pract 2004;10(6):368–74.

8. AVMA News. VMAT Helps to assess veterinary needs in Texas. American Veterinary Medical Association. 2011. Available at: https://www.avma.org/News/JAVMANews/Pages/s071501c.aspx. Accessed October 11, 2017.

9. Baker L, Thomassin PJ. Farm ownership and financial stress. Can J Agric Econ Can d'agroeconomie 1988;36:799–811.

10. Gerrard N. An application of a community psychology approach to dealing with farm stress. Can J Commun Ment Health 2000;19:89–100.
11. Keating NC. Reducing stress of farm men and women. Fam Relat 1987;36: 358–63.
12. Lunner-Kolstrup C, Kallioniemi MK, Lundqvist P, et al. International perspectives on psychosocial working conditions, mental health, and stress of dairy farm operators. J Agromedicine 2013;18(3):244–55.
13. McShane CJ, Quirk F. Mediating and moderating effects of work-home interference upon farm stresses and psychological distress. Aust J Rural Health 2009; 17(5):244–50.
14. Kubik W. The study of farm stress and coping: a critical evaluation (Order No. MQ30495). 1997.
15. Hood B, Seedsman T. Psychosocial investigation of individual and community responses to the experience of ovine Johne's disease in rural Victoria. Aust J Rural Health 2004;12:54–60.
16. Olff M, Koeter MWJ, Van Haaften EH, et al. Impact of a foot and mouth disease crisis on post-traumatic stress symptoms in farmers. Br J Psychiatry 2005;186:165–6.
17. Taylor MR, Agho KE, Stevens GJ, et al. Factors influencing psychological distress during a disease epidemic: data from Australia's first outbreak of equine influenza. BMC Public Health 2008;8:347.
18. Hanrahan C. Social work and human animal bonds and benefits in health research: a provincial study. Crit Soc Work 2013;14(1):63–79. Available at: http://www1.uwindsor.ca/criticalsocialwork/system/files/Hanrahan.pdf.
19. Perrin T. The business of urban animals survey: the facts and statistics on companion animals in Canada. Can Vet J 2009;50:48–52.
20. Serpell J. Animal assisted interventions in historical perspective. Handbook on Animal-Assisted therapy. 3rd edition 2010. p. 17–32.
21. Carmack BJ. The effects on family members and functioning after the death of a pet. Marriage Fam Rev 1985;8(3):149–61.
22. Clements PT, Benasutti KM, Carmone A. Support for bereaved owners of pets. Perspect Psychiatr Care 2003;39(2):49–54.
23. Packman W, Field NP, Carmack BJ, et al. Continuing bonds and psychosocial adjustment in pet loss. J Loss Trauma 2011;16(4):341–57.
24. Doka KJ. Disenfranchised grief. Bereave Care 1999;18(3):37–9.
25. Attig T. Disenfranchised grief revisited: discounting hope and love. Omega 2004; 49(3):197–215.
26. Cardeña E, Carlson E. Acute stress disorder revisited. Annu Rev Clin Psychol 2011;7:245–67.
27. Bryant RA. Acute stress disorder. Psychiatry 2006;5(7):238–9.
28. Gibson LE. Acute stress disorder. U.S. Department of Veterans Affairs. 2016. Available at: https://www.ptsd.va.gov/professional/treatment/early/acute-stress-disorder.asp. Accessed September 25, 2017.
29. Litz BT, Stein N, Delaney E, et al. Moral injury and moral repair in war veterans: a preliminary model and intervention strategy. Clin Psychol Rev 2009;29(8): 695–706.
30. Kavan MG, Elsasser GN, Barone EJ. The physician's role in managing acute stress disorder. Am Fam Physician 2012;86(7):643–9.
31. Phoenix Australia-Centre for Posttraumatic Mental health. Australian guidelines for the treatment of acute stress disorder & posttraumatic stress disorder. 2013. Available at: https://phoenixaustralia.org/wp-content/uploads/2015/03/Phoenix-ASD-PTSD-Guidelines.pdf. Accessed November 9, 2017.

32. Havron WS, Safcsak K, Loudon A, et al. Psychological effect of a mass casualty event on general surgery residents. J Surg Educ 2017;74(6):e74–80.
33. U.S. Department of Veteran Affairs. PTSD: National Center for PTSD. 2016. Available at: https://www.ptsd.va.gov/professional/materials/manuals/psych-first-aid.asp. Accessed November 9, 2017.
34. Ptacek J, Leonard K, McKee T. "I've Got Some Bad News...": veterinarians' recollections of communicating bad news to clients' J. J Appl Soc Psych 2004;34(2):366–90.
35. Ferguson C. "You can't do good medicine without good communication skills' 7 Actors and veterinarian-coaches help Vet Med students become great communicators. UToday. 2016. Available at: https://www.ucalgary.ca/utoday/issue/2016-02-16/you-cant-do-good-medicine-without-good-communication-skills. Accessed November 23, 2017.
36. Gunville L. Workshops bring mental health to forefront. WCVM Today. 2017. Available at: https://wcvmtoday.usask.ca/articles/2017/workshops-bring-mental-health-to-forefront.php. Accessed November 23, 2017.
37. Swisher RR, Elder GH, Lorenz FO, et al. The long arm of the farm: how an occupation structures exposure and vulnerability to stressors across role domains. J Health Soc Behav 1998;39(1):72.
38. Howe A, Smajdor A, Stöckl A. Towards an understanding of resilience and its relevance to medical training. Med Educ 2012;46(4):349–56.
39. Inglis-Rheinberger T. Provision of social support serves to farmers and rural communities in Canada. 2013. Available at: http://peifa.ca/wp-content/uploads/2014/06/Provision-of-social-support-services-to-farmers-and-rural-communities-in-Canada.pdf. Accessed August 30, 2017.
40. Wasson E. Wildfire support. Saskatoon. 2017.
41. U.S. Department of Health & Human Services. MentalHealth.gov Let's talk about it. Available at: https://www.mentalhealth.gov/. Accessed September 26, 2017.
42. Substance Abuse and Mental Health Services Administration. Find help & treatment. Available at: https://www.samhsa.gov/find-help. Accessed November 11, 2017.
43. The LifeLine Canada Foundation. Available at: https://thelifelinecanada.ca/help/crisis-centres/.
44. United Way Centraide Canada. 211. Available at: http://www.211.ca/.
45. American Veterinary Medical Association. Emergency preparedness and response. American Veterinary Medical Association. 2012. Available at: https://ebusiness.avma.org/files/productdownloads/emerg_prep_resp_guide.pdf. Accessed September 25, 2017.
46. Mellanby RJ. Incidence of suicide in the veterinary profession in England and Wales. Vet Rec 2005;157(14):415–7.
47. Platt B, Hawton K, Simkin S, et al. Suicidal behaviour and psychosocial problems in veterinary surgeons: a systematic review. Soc Psychiatry Psychiatr Epidemiol 2012;47(2):223–40.
48. Faragher T. Suicide in Australian veterinarians. Aust Vet J 2008;86(7):249.
49. Skipper GE, Williams JB. Failure to acknowledge high suicide risk among veterinarians. J Vet Med Educ 2012;39(1):79–82.
50. Wasson E. Consult for insowein piglet depopulation. Saskatoon; 2015.
51. American Veterinary Medical Association. Work and compassion fatigue. American Veterinary Medical Association. 2017. Available at: https://www.avma.org/ProfessionalDevelopment/Personal/PeerAndWellness/Pages/compassion-fatigue.aspx. Accessed November 23, 2017.

52. Maslach C, Schaufeli WB. Historical and conceptual development of burnout. In: Schaufeli WB, Maslach C, Marek T, editors. Series in applied psychology: social issues and questions. Professional burnout: Recent developments in theory and research. Philadelphia: Taylor & Francis; 1993. p. 1–16.
53. Smets EMA, Visser MRM, Oort FJ, et al. Perceived inequity: does it explain burnout among medical specialists?1. J Appl Soc Psychol 2004;34(9):1900–18.
54. Hunt MR, Schwartz L, Fraser V. "How far do you go and where are the issues surrounding that?" dilemmas at the boundaries of clinical competency in humanitarian health work. Prehosp Disaster Med 2013;28(5):502–8.
55. American Veterinary Medical Association. Self-care for veterinarians. American Veterinary Medical Association. 2017. Available at: https://www.avma.org/ProfessionalDevelopment/Personal/PeerAndWellness/Pages/self-care.aspx. Accessed November 23, 2017.
56. Hart L, Yamamoto M. Self-care for veterinarians. Merck manual veterinary manual. 2016. Available at: http://www.merckvetmanual.com/behavior/the-human-animal-bond/self-care-for-veterinarians. Accessed November 23, 2017.
57. World Health Organization. Self-care for health: a handbook for community health workers & volunteers. World Health Organization; 2013. Available at: http://apps.searo.who.int/PDS_DOCS/B5084.pdf.
58. Saskatchewan Veterinary Medical Association. SVMA member wellness program. 2017. Available at: http://www.svma.sk.ca/uploads/pdf/Wellness/Professional wellness program Nov 6-2017.pdf. Accessed November 23, 2017.
59. Nguyen AT, Trout KE, Chen LW, et al. Nebraska's rural behavioral healthcare workforce distribution and relationship between supply and county characteristics. Rural Remote Health 2016;16(2):3645.
60. Watanabe-Galloway S, Madison L, Watkins KL, et al. Recruitment and retention of mental health care providers in rural Nebraska: perceptions of providers and administrators. Rural Remote Health 2015;15(4):3392.
61. University of Tennessee College of Veterinary Medicine. Suicide awareness in veterinary education. Available at: https://vetmed.tennessee.edu/outreach/SAVE/Pages/default.aspx. Accessed October 11, 2017.
62. Association of American Veterinary Medical Colleges. Wellness modules added to zoetis' vetvance program. VetMedEducator. 2017. Available at: http://aavmc.org/VetMedEducatorDec2016.aspx. Accessed November 23, 2017.

# *Moving?*

## *Make sure your subscription moves with you!*

To notify us of your new address, find your **Clinics Account Number** (located on your mailing label above your name), and contact customer service at:

**Email: journalscustomerservice-usa@elsevier.com**

**800-654-2452** (subscribers in the U.S. & Canada)
**314-447-8871** (subscribers outside of the U.S. & Canada)

**Fax number: 314-447-8029**

**Elsevier Health Sciences Division
Subscription Customer Service
3251 Riverport Lane
Maryland Heights, MO 63043**

*To ensure uninterrupted delivery of your subscription, please notify us at least 4 weeks in advance of move.

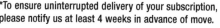

ELSEVIER

Printed and bound by CPI Group (UK) Ltd, Croydon, CR0 4YY

07/10/2024

01040500-0015